Can
I Just
Ask?

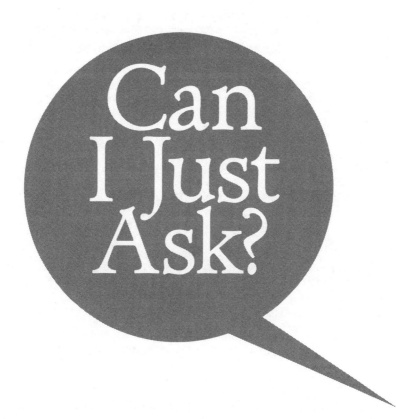

DR CHRISTIAN JESSEN

HAY HOUSE

Australia • Canada • Hong Kong • India
South Africa • United Kingdom • United States

First published and distributed in the United Kingdom by:
Hay House UK Ltd, 292B Kensal Rd, London W10 5BE. Tel.: (44) 20 8962 1230;
Fax: (44) 20 8962 1239. www.hayhouse.co.uk

Published and distributed in the United States of America by:
Hay House, Inc., PO Box 5100, Carlsbad, CA 92018-5100. Tel.: (1) 760 431 7695
or (800) 654 5126; Fax: (1) 760 431 6948 or (800) 650 5115.
www.hayhouse.com

Published and distributed in Australia by:
Hay House Australia Ltd, 18/36 Ralph St, Alexandria NSW 2015.
Tel.: (61) 2 9669 4299; Fax: (61) 2 9669 4144. www.hayhouse.com.au

Published and distributed in the Republic of South Africa by:
Hay House SA (Pty), Ltd, PO Box 990, Witkoppen 2068.
Tel./Fax: (27) 11 467 8904. www.hayhouse.co.za

Published and distributed in India by:
Hay House Publishers India, Muskaan Complex, Plot No.3, B-2, Vasant Kunj,
New Delhi – 110 070. Tel.: (91) 11 4176 1620; Fax: (91) 11 4176 1630.
www.hayhouse.co.in

Distributed in Canada by:
Raincoast, 9050 Shaughnessy St, Vancouver, BC V6P 6E5.
Tel.: (1) 604 323 7100; Fax: (1) 604 323 2600

The information given in this book should not be treated as a substitute for
professional medical advice; always consult a medical practitioner. Any use of
the information in this book is at the reader's discretion and risk. Neither the
author nor the publisher can be held responsible for any loss, claim or damage
arising out of the use, or misuse, or the suggestions made or the failure to take
medical advice.

A catalogue record for this book is available from the British Library.

ISBN 978-1-84850-246-8

Printed in the UK by CPI William Clowes Ltd, Beccles, NR34 7TL.

All of the papers used in this product are recyclable, and made from wood
grown in managed, sustainable forests and manufactured at mills certified to
ISO 14001 and/or EMAS.

Contents

Introduction

There is one constant about doctoring that is universally agreed upon by all medics: we are never, ever off duty. I don't mean that if someone collapses in the street we must go running to help, or if a passenger is taken ill on a plane we are obliged to go to their aid (though of course we are!). I mean in everyday life, during everyday conversations. Family gatherings all too often turn into mini-clinics, with brothers wanting to ask about this mole or that lump, aunts wanting info on which is the best HRT for them, and ever-wary grandparents wanting to check up on their own GP's competence in prescribing the correct blood pressure tablets. At nearly every conceivable occasion, once we have revealed our chosen trade, the questions quickly come rushing in – and by the hundreds, too. Dinner parties are definitely the worst. The more wine the guests drink, the bolder the questions get – things people have clearly been desperate to ask for years, but can only query under the liberating influence of wine and good food, never in the austere environs of their local GP surgery.

This got me thinking. Perhaps it would save us doctors a lot of breath if I collected together all the questions we get asked. Perhaps it would actually be a good reference book? After all, of whom can you ask all these questions? You can't make an appointment with your GP just to ask what your appendix does. Maybe your question seems just too silly to waste anyone's time over (*Does chewing gum really stay in your system for seven years if you swallow it?*). Perhaps the question is a little morbid and might cause raised eyebrows (*Do we poo ourselves when we die?*) or is just too buttock-clenchingly embarrassing to ask anyone, ever (*Why does my vaginal discharge smell so bad?*). The Internet contains vast amounts of information, but how do you know if the site you are looking at is accurate and up to date?

So I decided to put together this collection of the most common and curious questions that we doctors get asked. I sat down and talked with colleagues, and made notes of many of the things I get asked, both in the clinic and out. I went through old letters and emails, thought of every person who ever stopped me in the street or at a party with a question, and recalled as many drunken dinners as I could. I've even thrown in lots of top 10 lists and boxes of interesting facts and figures to keep you hungry for more.

So now you don't have to ask anyone out loud, and you can let us docs forget about medicine and allow us to enjoy our dinners out, free to gossip about *The X Factor* and not X chromosomes, because it's all here instead, divided neatly into sections to help you find the answer to your particular mystery. It covers male and female problems, sex, diet and fitness, and even some oddities that I couldn't fit into a conventional pigeonhole (*Will I get arthritis if I crack my knuckles?*). If you have a certain condition and want to find out more, or just want to know some extraordinary facts about your body, this is the book for you.

I have also become increasingly aware of the considerable number of myths circulating around, mistakenly advising that such-and-such a behaviour is guaranteed to improve health. I'm sure many are recommended in good faith, but medicine has come a long way and we really shouldn't be propagating this sort of nonsense any longer. The advice that you drink two litres of water a day, avoid carbohydrates if you want to lose weight, detox regularly and try homoeopathy are just some of the 21st-century health mantras that are often unquestioningly accepted – and in my view are pure hokum – so I cover as many of these as I can, too. And don't get me started about chiropractors ...

Dr Christian Jessen
London 2010
www.drchristianjessen.com

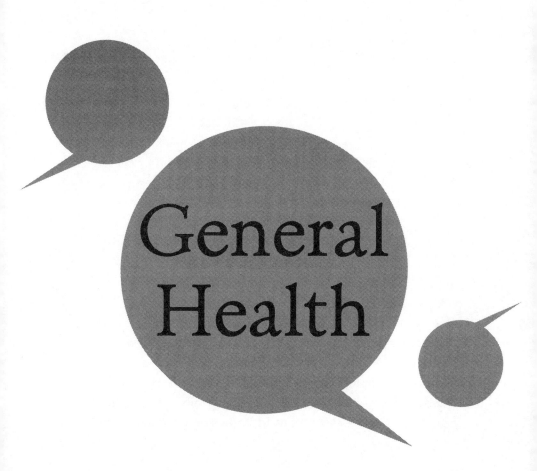

Should you really feed a cold? And if so, why is chicken soup always recommended?

Eating not only helps your body to combat a cold, but can also help you feel better. Dutch researchers have found that eating stimulates the very type of immune response that destroys the viruses that cause colds. Their experiments showed that six hours after we eat a meal, our levels of *gamma interferon* – a substance produced by infection-fighting cells and involved in the process by which T cells destroy cells attacked by a foreign invader (pathogen) – increase fourfold. By contrast, gamma interferon levels actually drop in people who drink only water when they have a cold.

Not just any old food will do, though. You need to choose a healthy, balanced diet. Chicken soup has been offered to the bed-bound since the dawn of time, and it seems the gesture is not at all futile. The soup has anti-inflammatory properties, and some studies have shown that it can reduce the movement of the white blood cells that can cause congestion and other undesirable cold symptoms.

What about starving a fever?

Most doctors would advise you to stick to a normal diet whether you have a fever or not. Some research even suggests that fasting during an illness may be dangerous. As we learned from the question above, restricting food intake hinders the immune system's ability to respond to an infection, because it deprives key cells of the energy they need to produce proteins that recognize invaders and target them for destruction.

Did You Know... Your hearing is less acute after a large meal. Musicians and singers often avoid eating before a concert for this very reason.

Why do we have earwax? And what is the best way to remove it?

Earwax is a useful substance that your body produces to protect and clean the ears. It has a number of important functions: it cleans, lubricates and protects the lining of your ear by trapping dirt and repelling water. It is also slightly acidic and has antibacterial properties. Without earwax, the skin inside your ear may become dry, cracked and infected, or waterlogged and sore.

The rate of earwax production is usually fairly steady, but if you get colds or have a lot of allergies then you may produce more. It can build up and become blocked, which will affect your hearing. People have one of two types of earwax: dry or wet; it is the wet type that can get blocked up. Never use cotton buds, as they just push the wax further into your ears and impact it. Forget those ear candle things, too; they will do nothing except drip hot wax on you. Chewing gum can help shift it (by chewing it, not sticking it in your ear), and olive oil in the ear will soften it and help it work its way out.

When I fly I get sharp pains in my ear. They usually go away quite quickly afterwards but my hearing can be a bit muffled for a while after. Why does this happen, and what can I do about it?

When you go up and down in a plane you experience considerable pressure changes within your ears. These changes usually affect you more when the tubes connecting your ears and nose are blocked due to a cold or infection.

I suggest you try some nasal drops one hour before you take the flight, and when you are landing chew gum or some toffee so that you keep swallowing. Swallowing helps open the tubes and clears the pressure, and so relieves the pain. Opening your mouth really wide, as when you yawn, can help, too. You could consider having a check-up to see if you have any chronic infections or sinusitis.

I can see blood in my urine. What should I do?

Get yourself checked by a doctor. The commonest cause of this is an infection, but there are other causes: kidney stones or bladder stones, and even growths in the bladder. The important thing to say is that it is never 'normal'. It is a sign that something is wrong and needs looking into. Infections can be simply treated with an antibiotic, but you definitely need to report this to your GP who will want, at the very least, to send off a sample of your urine to the lab. Some 4 per cent of the population have blood in their urine without any detectable cause, but it tends not to be visible to the eye. It's more likely to be found on 'dipstick' testing. Visible blood in the urine should always be investigated. Remember that some foods, like beetroot, can colour your urine pink. Alarming, but entirely harmless.

I have a small hard lump growing on the back of my hand. It's been there for a while – what could it be?

This sounds like a really common thing called a *ganglion*, which is a little jelly-filled cyst that grows around tendons, which is why the back of the hand is a common place to get them. It's not serious at all and can be left well alone. The historical treatment was to whack them really hard with a big book, like a bible, to burst them, but I don't recommend you try this! If it is sore or causing problems, then a doctor can put a needle in it to drain it, or it can be removed surgically. Otherwise just leave it alone as it may just disappear in time.

Did You Know... Only around one-third of the human race has perfect vision, and this proportion decreases significantly with increasing age.

I am suffering from two groin hernias. I keep being told that I need to lose weight, but what can I do that won't make them worse?

Most hernias are caused by increased pressure in the abdomen, caused by straining (as when lifting heavy objects), coughing, or if constipated. If you are overweight then this will also contribute, because much of the excess fat tissue is deposited around the intestine inside the abdomen, increasing the pressure on the tummy muscles and forcing the intestine to protrude through any weakness in the abdominal wall – a hernia. Groin hernias are the most common in men because of a natural weakness there, left when the testicles descend into the scrotum before or after birth.

You need to keep your weight down to prevent the hernia getting worse, and also to make surgery easier. Exercises to avoid are any involving heavy lifting, pulling or pushing, as these involve closing off your throat, which only serves to increase abdominal pressure and the size of the hernia. I suggest that the best thing to do would be aerobic-type exercise, for 30 minutes at a time, every other day. The best ones are swimming and using an exercise bike.

I have varicose veins on my legs. Will exercising make them even worse?

No, exercise will not make your varicose veins worse. In fact, it should actually improve the circulation through your legs, so may make the varicose veins less noticeable. Blood goes into your legs through your arteries, and returns to the heart through your veins. Your veins have valves in them to stop the blood going the wrong way, and varicose veins occur when the valves in your veins don't work properly and the veins distend and stretch. If they are particularly unsightly or painful, then you can have an operation to have them removed.

My mum and my grandma have osteoporosis and I'm worried that I'll get it, too. I'm 26 and want to know what I can do to avoid it.

Osteoporosis is a condition where your bones become thin and weak, and can break easily. It can happen to women after the menopause because of changes to their hormone levels, which normally regulate calcium levels and bone strength.

To avoid osteoporosis, the best first step is to look to your diet. Calcium-rich foods like green veg, nuts and soy products are all good. Dairy and fish are also good sources. If you think you aren't getting enough and don't have much dairy in your diet either, then you could take a supplement with calcium and vitamin D.

The other important thing for keeping your bones strong is weight-bearing exercise. The more you can do now, while you are young, the stronger your bones will be as you get older. Try walking, jogging, skipping, weight-training or aerobics, and keep your body weight within a healthy range, because being very underweight will put you at risk, too.

Did You Know... We all have our own unique smell, except for identical twins. Newborn babies can recognize the smell of their mothers, and many of us can pinpoint the smell of our significant others and those we are close to. Part of that smell is determined by genetics, but it's also largely determined by environment, diet and personal hygiene products, all of which create a unique chemistry for each of us.

I have lost my sense of smell. I can't remember any event that caused it, and it is really spoiling my enjoyment of food, as I can't taste it properly. What could be causing it?

Loss of smell needs to be taken seriously, so it's important that the cause is found. The most common causes are nose infections, colds and hay fever. They only cause a temporary loss of smell, however, and it should come back when the problem settles.

Some women can lose their sense of smell because of an underactive thyroid gland, and this problem can be revealed by blood tests. It can be corrected with tablets to correct the lack of thyroid hormone. The most sinister cause is a brain tumour pushing on the smell nerves in the top of your nose. Although this is rare you must have tests to exclude this possibility. I would go to your GP as soon as you can and get started with the investigations.

I have recently had an operation on my tummy. What can I do to make the scar smaller and less noticeable?

If your scar is relatively new, then it will be quite dark and prominent, which is normal. Scars do settle down and fade with time, although this can take between six months and a year. The good news is that there are products available to help if you can't wait that long. You can get silicon gel patches that you stick over the scar, or a silicon-based cream called Dermatix that you need to rub on the scar twice a day. They take a few months to work and are expensive, but can be effective, especially with scars from burns (for which they are often used in hospitals). A simpler and cheaper solution for you may be to try Bio-Oil® or vitamin E capsules. Cut them open and massage the oil into the scar every day. This will help it heal and become much more discreet.

When I get nervous I get big red blotches over my face, neck, chest and arms that are very noticeable. Drinking makes them worse. Is there is anything I can take to stop them appearing?

You have a condition called idiopathic craniofacial erythema, or excess blushing, which seems to affect up to 10 per cent of the population. It's caused by the blood vessels in your skin dilating due to chemical and nerve signals that occur when you get stressed or pressured. It can be difficult to treat, but there has been lots of success with cognitive behavioural therapy (CBT) and neuro-linguistic programming (NLP). There is also an operation available to cut the nerves that control blushing. This has its risks, of course, but can work well for some.

Did You Know... If something cannot be dissolved in saliva, then it cannot be tasted. For foods – or anything else – to have a taste, chemicals from the substance must be dissolved by saliva in order to stimulate the taste buds.

I have really bad breath, and have done for years. It seems to come from the back of my mouth/tongue. Can you get antibiotics to reduce the amount of bacteria in the mouth, and would this be worth a try?

Bad breath is a problem that can affect everyone at some stage or other. We all know what it's like getting close to someone after a meal of garlic and onions. Your case sounds a little more serious, however. I suggest that the first thing you do is to get a full dental check-up, as gum disease and tooth decay are some of the main culprits, along with cigarette smoking and excess boozing.

Dieting can also make your breath bad – the Atkins diet being a notorious example of this. Other possibilities include liver or kidney disease, and even some drugs, such as antidepressants, which reduce the amount of saliva produced. Make sure you floss your teeth regularly, and it may be worth investing in a tongue scraper – although, be warned: the colour and smell of what you remove when you first use it will probably horrify you!

If you have tried all these and none works, then it is possible that you may have an overgrowth of bacteria in your mouth, which will need an antibiotic called Metronidazole to get rid of. You will need to get a prescription from your GP.

Is Botox safe?

Everyone has heard of Botox, but not everyone knows that it is actually a purified form of the toxin made by bacteria that causes food poisoning! However, injected into facial lines, it temporarily paralyses the contractions of the underlying muscles, which, in turn, reduces the appearance of wrinkles.

There are very few risks associated with Botox injections, but I would only recommend that a trained doctor administer it because a good knowledge of facial anatomy is needed to achieve a satisfactory result and results can vary according to the practitioner. The effects aren't permanent – they last only up to six months – so be prepared to need a top-up later on, and remember, as with most cosmetic procedures, less is more.

What exactly is Bell's palsy?

The muscles of the face are controlled by the facial nerve, which comes out of a hole in the skull just below and in front of the ear. From there it spreads like a fan across the face, with branches going to each of the many tiny muscles that control our facial expressions. Damage to this nerve causes all these facial muscles to stop working, which shows in affected patients as an inability to smile or close one eye properly.

By far the most common cause of this type of paralysis is Bell's palsy, caused by an inflammation of the facial nerve as it leaves the skull. The exact reason for this inflammation, and subsequent paralysis, is unknown. When the condition starts, the patient develops a sudden paralysis of the face muscles on one side only. There may be some mild to moderate pain at the point where the nerve leaves the skull beside the ear, but this settles after a few days. There may also be a disturbance to taste sensation. Two-thirds of patients recover completely within a few weeks with no treatment. Most of the others obtain partial recovery, but 10 per cent are significantly affected by facial paralysis for the long term.

Is all this stuff about it being dangerous and cancer-causing to live near electricity pylons true? Has there actually been any research done on it?

There is research being done, and a lot of it is still ongoing. The UK Childhood Cancer Study concluded there was 'no evidence that exposure to magnetic fields associated with the electricity supply in the UK increases risks for childhood leukaemia, cancers of the central nervous system, or any other childhood cancer'. But scientists at the World Health Organization criticized this research, saying that it was incomplete: not all forms of exposure were measured, and only small numbers of children in the higher-exposure categories were used. This makes the reassurance that the UK Childhood Cancer Study tried to give a little hard to swallow. I would say that the jury is still out on this one.

Did You Know... Small noises cause the pupils of your eyes to dilate. This is almost certainly why loud, uninvited noises can so disturb people doing close work, like surgeons and watchmakers. The sound causes their pupils to change focus and blurs their vision, making it harder to do their job.

Every now and then I get a weird twitching in the muscles of my eyelid. It feels like it's jumping a bit. What causes this?

This is a really common symptom and often occurs during periods of stress or fatigue. We don't really know the exact cause, but we do know it is of no significance and is certainly not a sign of any sinister underlying brain or neurological disease. It is more likely to be a sign that you need a good night's sleep. While there is no proof that caffeine makes it worse, decreasing caffeine consumption is said to help some people.

Eyelid twitching is not the same as a spasm of the muscles around the eye that causes it to close. Called blepharospasm, this should precipitate a trip to your doctor's.

Top 10 Unnecessary Body Parts

1) Tonsils

These are a part of the body we can certainly manage very well without, and which can cause some people a lot of pain due to chronic inflammation. Tonsils are lymphoid tissues that are prone to becoming infected and swelling up. Some people believe they should not be removed, as they may be involved with our immune system's development.

2) Adenoids

These strange glands are masses of lymphoid tissue located at the very back of the nose. They are part of your childhood immune system that trap inhaled bacteria and viruses. As you age, your adenoids shrink, making them useless in adulthood.

3) Sinuses

Sinuses are one part of the body about which not much is known. They're nothing but air-filled spaces, but we have many in our heads. Some say that they insulate our eyes, while others suggest that they influence our voice's tone and pitch. No one knows exactly what they're for, but we do know that they can become infected and cause headaches.

4) Male nipples

These don't really need much explanation, I suspect. Males don't breastfeed, so nipples really aren't needed. For us guys they are merely decorative.

5) Wisdom teeth

Your wisdom teeth are located at the back of your mouth. They were once very helpful, especially when humans had a diet that consisted of a lot of tough meat, as they allowed us to chew our food properly. Nowadays, many people don't even get them, and if they do the teeth can grow in the wrong way and cause pain, meaning they are often removed.

6) Coccyx

Also known as the tailbone, this is the last part of the human vertebrae. It is made up of five separate or fused vertebrae and is the remnant of our vestigial tail. To be fair it is not entirely useless, as it acts as the point of attachment for many different ligaments, tendons and muscles. But generally the coccyx is much more important in mammals with tails than in humans.

7) Gallbladder

This is a small organ used to store bile, which aids digestion. Stones can form within it causing pain, nausea, indigestion and infections, and as we can function perfectly well without one, it is often removed surgically.

8) Appendix

This is one I get asked about frequently. One purpose of the appendix, we think, is to digest cellulose. It was a more important and necessary organ when the human diet consisted mostly of plants. Today it is not so necessary, and its presence is usually made known only when it becomes infected and inflamed.

9) Plica semilunaris

Otherwise known as your third eyelid. Yes, you do have three, but it's one of the many body parts that we don't need. If you pull each of your eyelids up, the plica semilunaris will be exposed. It's this part that produces 'sleep dust', that crust occurring in the corners of your eyes after waking.

10) Errector Pili

The truly defunct nature of these is, I agree, debatable. The errector pili are extremely small muscle fibres that are attached to each hair follicle on your body, which when contracted make your hairs stand on end and cause goosebumps. They are really only useful in animals with much more hair because they provide a layer of insulation and can make animals look much larger when threatened.

Is it true that you are more at risk of heart disease if you have bad teeth?

This is a subject that researchers have been studying for years. We know that bacteria from the mouth can get into the bloodstream during dental procedures and cause serious heart infections in people with heart defects or artificial valves. But more recently, multiple studies have shown connections between gum disease and heart disease. They include links between higher rates of periodontitis, tooth loss and other oral problems to increased risk factors for coronary artery disease, thickened carotid arteries and other types of cardiovascular disease. The observations made so far are that the rate of heart disease increases with the number of teeth patients are missing, that intensive treatment of periodontal disease may reverse atherosclerosis (hardening of the arteries), and that people exposed to certain bacteria associated with gum disease also have an increased risk of cardiovascular disease. There may be a simple explanation: perhaps people with bad teeth simply lead less healthy lifestyles, so it's not the bad teeth causing the heart disease, but the bad lifestyle.

Heart disease has numerous risk factors, some of which are beyond your control. Your dental health is up to you, however, so it's worth bearing in mind that keeping your teeth and gums healthy may also help your heart.

What exactly is ME? Does it really exist, or is it just another modern-day made-up condition invented by people who feel tired all the time?

ME stands for myalgic encephalomyelitis, otherwise known as chronic fatigue syndrome. It's one of a number of diseases categorized as post-viral syndromes. Remarkably little is known about them. In some people a viral infection like flu can be followed by a chronic inflammation of many organs of the body, causing aches and pains and tiredness.

The symptoms of ME vary hugely from one patient to another, and include arthritis, muscle pains, headaches, nausea, vomiting, diarrhoea, skin rashes, abdominal cramps, depression, mood changes and severe tiredness. Women are affected five times more often than men. Most people have the disease for many months or a few years, and it then slowly fades away.

There are no tests that can confirm a diagnosis of chronic fatigue syndrome. Everything in sufferers appears completely normal except for the fact that they are so tired that they cannot perform their normal daily activities. It is therefore known as a diagnosis of exclusion.

Because we don't know what causes chronic fatigue syndrome, we don't know how to treat it. There are as many theories and treatments as there are doctors, and every alternative therapist – from osteopaths to naturopaths – seems to claim that they can cure the problem. I only know that antidepressant and anti-inflammatory medications seem to be the best options currently available.

Did You Know... You are born with eyes that are the same size as when you are an adult – they never grow. Your nose and ears never stop growing, however, and research has shown that their growth peaks in seven-year cycles.

Do earlobe creases really indicate you may have coronary heart disease?

An earlobe crease is a line that runs diagonally right across the earlobe, to its lower tip. Its status as a portent of heart trouble has been abundantly confirmed. A Swedish study of 520 autopsies found that the presence of earlobe creases had a 'positive predictive value' for coronary artery disease of 68 per cent, and 80 per cent in the under-forties. A Turkish study found that they are a higher risk factor for heart disease than diabetes, family history of cardiovascular trouble, or smoking. Of 340 patients admitted to the Montreal Heart Institute, 91 per cent of those with earlobe creases had heart disease, versus 61 per cent of those without. Put simply, not having a crease doesn't necessarily mean you don't have heart disease, but if you do have one, then it's a pretty good bet you do.

Other predictive factors for heart disease include having a short ring finger, male pattern baldness, gum disease and dry earwax. Some of the research behind this is less than convincing, however. If you have one of these, don't panic, it doesn't mean that a heart attack is inevitable and unavoidable, just that you may need to pay a little more attention to your heart health.

Did You Know... By the age of 60, most people will have lost about half their taste buds. Older people tend to lose their ability to taste, and many find that they need much stronger flavourings in order to be able to appreciate their food.

Can air injected into the bloodstream really kill you? I have to assume it's the reason for tapping on a syringe to get the air out of it. Is it any amount of air, or does it have to be quite a lot?

An air embolism, the medical term for air in the bloodstream, can definitely kill you. How it does this depends on the size of the air bubble and where it lodges in your body.

You mention air entering accidentally via an injection or IV tube, but it can also enter when blood vessels are cut during surgery, and during ascent after scuba diving, where an increase in air volume in the lungs pushes tiny bubbles of air into the bloodstream, which expand as you rise. A more bizarre route involves blowing air into the vagina of a pregnant woman during oral sex.

A small amount can block capillaries in vital organs, most seriously in the brain, causing anything from pain and inflammation to neurological damage and paralysis. A big bubble can stop blood flow through your heart, and even stop the heart itself.

Emboli from injections or IVs are typically confined to veins, but if a bubble ends up in your arteries then it can block your coronary arteries or the blood supply to your brain. The former type of blockage can mean death.

How much air is needed to kill you? Generally speaking, it's quite a lot. One journal declared that 300 millilitres can be lethal, but it's said that serious damage can result from as little as 20 millilitres. Neither is a very small amount.

By way of a grim tale, after public outcry stopped the Nazis gassing mental patients, psychiatric institutions were ordered to continue so-called 'mercy killings' by less conspicuous means, namely by injection with air, which usually killed the patients within minutes.

Is it true that sleep before midnight is more important than sleep after midnight?

My mother always told me this, but I suspect it was just a ruse to get me to go to bed earlier. It didn't work. Now that I am older and dare to argue with her more, I can say that there is nothing particularly special about sleep before midnight. Upon falling asleep at any time, most people go through a 90-minute cycle of non-REM sleep followed by REM sleep, and the ratio of non-REM-to-REM sleep changes across the night: the earlier in the night, the greater the propensity for deep non-REM sleep, and the later in the morning, the greater the propensity for REM sleep. This means an early-to-bed person will have a sleep pattern that is biased towards more non-REM sleep, and dream less. Is this better? Who can say?

Did You Know... By 60 years of age, 60 per cent of men and 40 per cent of women will snore. Normal snores average at around 60 decibels, the noise level of normal speech; intense snores can reach more than 80 decibels, the approximate level caused by a pneumatic drill breaking up concrete.

I get a lot of headaches and am terrified that I have a brain tumour. I have seen my GP about this but he just dismisses my concerns. How can he be so sure I don't have a tumour?

Let me introduce you to a 14th-century logician and Franciscan friar called William of Ockham, who is credited with a principle known as 'Occam's razor'. He suggested that 'entities should not be multiplied unnecessarily.' Actually he wrote it in a much longer form in Latin, but I have translated for you. The most useful interpretation of the principle for scientists is 'when you have two competing theories that make exactly the same predictions, the simpler one is the better.' Or, put even more simply: 'common things are common.'

There is a popular medical adage that paraphrases this: 'when you hear hoofbeats, think horses, not zebras.' It means that a common condition is probably more likely to be responsible for a patient's symptoms than a very rare one. And so, back to your original question: headaches are common, brain tumours are rare. The most common causes of headaches are tension headaches, migraines, sinusitis and trapped nerves. High blood pressure does not give you headaches, as is often believed. Poor, uncorrected vision can also be responsible.

Just for the sake of completeness, the warning signs of brain tumours include pain that is worst in the morning and then improves as the day progresses, early-morning vomiting, neurological problems, loss of vision and clumsiness. Your GP will, I hope, have taken your symptoms into full consideration, and made his pronouncement based on these facts. And he is probably right.

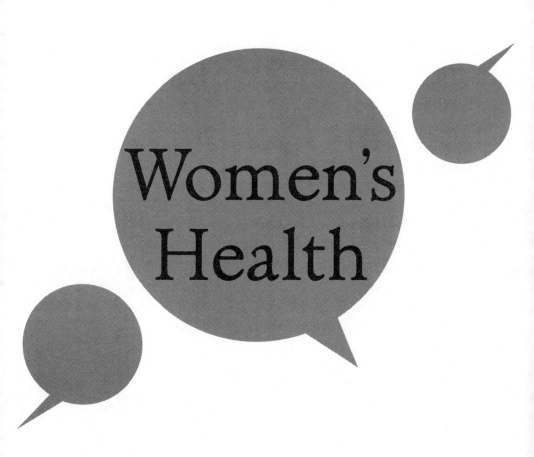

I get really bad attacks of thrush in the winter, and over-the-counter creams don't help at all. What else can I try?

Thrush is caused by a yeast called *Candida albicans* that is often present on the skin without causing any problems. If conditions on the skin change, however, then it can start to grow and cause problems. Warm, wet, airless places are perfect for it to grow in, so try to avoid wearing tight synthetic clothes and underwear, and also stop using strong soaps and detergents. If you have any problems with your immune system or you have been taking antibiotics, you may also get attacks of thrush. Being on the Pill and having diabetes also increase your chances of suffering recurrent thrush infections. Go for a general health check-up with your GP and ask for a stronger treatment: Canesten tablets or pessaries may be more effective for you. Remember that there are other types of infections that could cause your symptoms and that may require different treatments, so if this is an ongoing problem, a swab could be taken and assessed in a lab.

I have been told that I have got genital warts and that they can give women cancer – is this true, and what can I do to stop them?

Warts are one of the most common sexually acquired infections. In fact, you don't actually have to have had sex with someone to catch warts, although genital warts are most often acquired through sexual contact. A virus, of which there are about a hundred different types, causes them. If you had verrucas as a child, then you have had warts. It is true that there are certain strains of the virus which, over a long period of time, can cause changes to the cells of your cervix which may lead to cervical cancer developing if left undetected and untreated. This is nothing to worry about, however, as there is an effective NHS screening process in place to look for these early changes. If you have never had a smear test, then I suggest you go for one, and then keep them up every three years. You don't need to do any more than this if the results are normal.

Did You Know... Women's hearts beat faster than men's.

I have funny spots on my breasts. They are small lumps around my nipple and sometimes produce white pus when squeezed. They never seem to go away like spots do. What are they?

What you are describing sounds like little things called Montgomery's tubercles, and you can rest assured that they are completely normal. They are basically tiny sebaceous glands which all women have in varying numbers. Some have only one or two while others have nearer 30 or more. I doubt what you are seeing coming out of them is pus. Montgomery's tubercles secrete small amounts of a lubricating substance, which maintains the skin's pH and keeps it healthy; it will be this substance that you are squeezing out of them. They can become more prominent during pregnancy and while breastfeeding. As long as there is no pain, redness or swelling, then they are nothing to worry about. Try not to squeeze them, as you could cause them to become infected.

I'm a 32-year-old lesbian but I am still a virgin. Do I need to go for a smear test? I keep getting called for one by my GP.

Any woman of any age can develop cervical cancer, so in theory every woman over the age of 20 should have a cervical smear test. But as long as you are a non-smoker (smoking increases your risk of cervical cancer), then you are in one of the lower risk categories for developing cervical cancer. This is because we know your risk of cervical cancer increases with the number of male sexual partners you have had, and also if you started having sex at a young age. These factors clearly do not apply to you. If you have never had sex with a male partner then you probably don't need to have a cervical smear test. Unless you have a strong family history of cervical cancer or you have symptoms such as bleeding between your periods, then it isn't essential to have the test, because the risk of your developing cervical cancer is really low.

I get bad symptoms when I'm on my period. I'm about to go away for a really special holiday and want to know if it is possible to delay my period so it doesn't spoil things.

It certainly is possible to do this, and many women do so to avoid having a period over their wedding and honeymoon. If you are already taking the contraceptive pill, then you can avoid having your period while on your holiday by taking one packet back-to-back with another one, missing out the last seven blank pills or pill-free days. This will give you six weeks or so without a bleed. I suggest that you then go back to taking the Pill as normal to avoid the lining of your womb building up to unsatisfactory levels. Ask your GP for details to make sure you get it right.

If you're not currently on the Pill, then you can ask your GP for a medicine called norethisterone, which can be started three days before a period is due. You take it for the next seven days (when your period is due) and then stop it, at which time normal vaginal bleeding will take place. Norethisterone only needs to be taken as needed, whereas the Pill really needs to be started one to two months before, to be most effective.

Did You Know... Women blink twice as many times as men do. That's a lot of blinking every day. The average person, man or woman, blinks about 13 times a minute.

Can a hard knock on the breast give you breast cancer? I hit my breast playing sport and now have a hard lump there.

This is another of those great myths that do the rounds, usually among young women. There is no connection between breast cancer and injury or trauma to the breasts. It won't make a cancer occur, and nor will it increase your risk of getting one in any way, so don't worry. An injury may cause bruising and fibrous scar tissue to develop, which may explain the lump you feel. Fat necrosis is a rare benign breast condition that occurs when fatty breast tissue swells or becomes tender. It can occur when large-breasted women decide they are going to take up jogging without an adequately supportive bra – and the bouncing of the breasts causes tissue damage and injury. Fat necrosis could possibly be mistaken for a tumour on mammogram, but any symptoms it causes usually settle within a month.

Is there anything I can do to make my periods a little more bearable?

Some women suffer terribly each month from the symptoms of PMT. But there are tried-and-tested things that can make these symptoms less severe.

The first is to try to de-stress. Stress can make the symptoms of PMT much worse, so try to make a special effort to relax before and during your time of the month, as this can make a real difference.

Keep your weight within the normal healthy range. Losing too much can have an adverse effect on your menstrual cycle, causing abnormal bleeding or missed periods.

Try a zinc-rich diet. A diet low in zinc can exacerbate the cramps and bloating caused by menstruation. The best food sources of zinc are seafood, lean beef, lentils, wholegrain cereals, and liver and kidney.

The essential fats omega 3 and omega 6 have been clinically proven to reduce painful periods and help relieve the symptoms of PMT. Cold-water fish such as salmon, tuna, halibut and herring are the best sources of these two highly beneficial fatty acids.

Finally, research has shown that a regular workout can significantly reduce the symptoms of PMT. Even a ten-minute walk, three times a week, can dramatically ease the pain and discomfort of your period. Your GP will also have an arsenal of prescription medications that can be of help if you are still suffering.

Did You Know... Women can differentiate between more different smells than men can, and they remain better 'smellers' over their lifetimes. Studies have shown that women are also more able to identify exactly what a smell is than men. Some 2 per cent of the population have no sense of smell at all.

I pee during sex! It often happens near orgasm, and it's so humiliating that I am starting to avoid having sex because of it. What causes it and what can be done?

Despite the understandable embarrassment that you feel when it happens, it probably occurs to more women, more often than you may imagine. There are varying degrees of the problem, but most women only pee a very small volume – a teaspoonful or so. It occurs because the nerves in your bladder mistakenly tell your brain that it is the right time to pee, even if you don't need to or, obviously, particularly want to. It may be an explanation for the legend of female ejaculation. It's not really a medical problem as such, but there are some things you can try which may help.

Don't drink too much in the hours leading up to sex, particularly tea, coffee and alcohol. If possible, go for a pee immediately before you have sex, and finally, try to avoid sexual positions where you can feel increased pressure on your bladder due to the angle of penetration.

If the problem is severe or occurring at other times, too, then see your doctor to ask about incontinence medications, which can be taken just before sex. This should help you. Don't feel embarrassed to ask about this, as you really won't be the only one by any means.

Does having a coil really increase your chances of getting ovarian cysts, and if so, why? Can they turn into cancer or affect your fertility?

Ovarian cysts are fluid-filled sacs that occur inside or on the surface of the ovaries. The most common type is called a *functional cyst*. Every month as an egg is getting ready to be released, it is contained in a small cyst-like structure called a follicle. Usually this follicular sac breaks open and releases the egg, but sometimes the sac doesn't break open and continues to fill with fluid. Normally the fluid in these cysts is reabsorbed into the body in time, but sometimes it can continue to collect until the cysts are so large they cause pain or discomfort.

Sometimes the ovaries can become polycystic when each month the follicle doesn't break open. The female cycle continues as normal until eventually there can be many small cysts on each ovary. These can be painful and prevent normal conception from occurring, affecting your fertility. In some instances the cysts can be harmful. There is a possibility that they can be cancerous or that the fluid contained within them may hold some cancer cells.

There is one type of 'coil' called the Mirena coil, a progestogen-releasing intrauterine coil that does, indeed, increase your risk of having an ovarian cyst. Studies have shown this, but most of the resulting cysts are relatively small and cause no symptoms, and they usually resolve without treatment. They have been diagnosed in about 12 per cent of women using Mirena. However,

I should say that it is also much more effective than other coils, and avoids many of the side-effects that put women off this form of contraception.

10 Strange Psychiatric Conditions

1) Stockholm Syndrome
A psychological response sometimes seen in hostages, in which they show signs of sympathy, loyalty or even love for their captor, regardless of the risk in which they have been placed. The syndrome is also seen in situations of wife-beating, rape and child abuse. It takes its name from a bank robbery that occurred in Stockholm, in which the robbers held bank employees hostage for six days. The hostages became emotionally attached to the robbers and even defended their captors after they were freed from their six-day ordeal, refusing to testify against them.

2) Lima Syndrome
The exact opposite of Stockholm syndrome, this involves the hostage-takers becoming more sympathetic to the plights and needs of their hostages. Named after the Japanese embassy hostage crisis in Lima, Peru where 14 members of the Tupac Amaru Revolutionary Movement took hundreds of people hostage at a party at the official residence of Japan's ambassador to Peru. Within a few days the militants had released most of the captives, with seeming disregard for their importance, including the future president of Peru and the mother of the current president, and treated them all with utmost kindness and reverence.

3) Diogenes Syndrome
Diogenes was an ancient Greek philosopher who lived in a wine barrel and promoted ideas of nihilism and animalism. When he was asked by Alexander the Great what he wanted most in the world, he replied, 'For you to get out of my sunlight.' This condition is characterized by extreme self-neglect, reclusive tendencies and compulsive hoarding, sometimes of animals. It is found mainly in old people and is associated with senile breakdown.

4) Paris Syndrome

Paris syndrome is a condition exclusive to Japanese tourists and nationals, which causes them to have a mental breakdown while visiting Paris. Millions of Japanese tourists visit the city every year, and around 20 of them suffer this illness and have to be returned home. The condition is essentially a severe form of 'culture shock'. Japanese tourists who come to the city are unable to reconcile their idyllic view of it, seen in films, with the reality of a modern, bustling metropolis. The Japanese embassy in Paris has a 24-hour hotline for tourists suffering from severe culture shock, and can provide emergency hospital treatment if necessary.

5) Stendhal Syndrome

A psychosomatic illness that causes rapid heartbeat, dizziness, confusion and even hallucinations when an individual is exposed to art, usually when the art is particularly 'beautiful' or a large amount of art is in a single place. The term can also be used to describe a similar reaction to a surfeit of choice in other circumstances, for example when confronted with immense beauty in the natural world. Traditionally sufferers would have been described as being of a rather sensitive nature.

6) Jerusalem Syndrome

This is the name given to a group of mental phenomena involving the presence of either religiously themed obsessive ideas, delusions or other psychosis-like experiences that are triggered by, or lead to, a visit to the city of Jerusalem. It emerges while in the city and causes psychotic delusions, which tend to dissipate after a few weeks. All the people who have suffered this spontaneous psychosis have had a history of previous mental illness.

7) Capgras Delusion

A rare disorder in which a person holds a delusional belief that an identical-looking impostor has replaced a spouse or other close family member. It's most common in patients with schizophrenia, although it can occur in people with dementia, or those who have suffered a brain injury.

8) Fregoli Delusion

This is the exact opposite of the Capgras delusion. It's a rare disorder in which a person holds a delusional belief that different people are in fact a single person who changes appearance or uses multiple disguises. It was first reported in 1927 by two psychiatrists who discussed the case study of a 27-year-old woman who believed that she was being persecuted by two actors taking the form of all the people she knew or met.

9) Reduplicative Paramnesia

The delusional belief that a place or location has been duplicated, existing in two or more places simultaneously, or that it has been 'relocated' to another site. For example, a person may believe that he is in fact not in the hospital to which he was admitted, but in an identical-looking hospital in a different part of the country. The term was first used in 1903 by the Czechoslovakian neurologist Arnold Pick to describe a condition in a patient with suspected Alzheimer's disease who insisted that she had been moved from Pick's city clinic to one she claimed looked identical but was in a familiar suburb.

10) Amputee Identity Disorder

A neurological and psychological disorder in which sufferers have a feeling that they would be happier living life as an amputee. It is usually accompanied by the desire to amputate one or more of their healthy limbs in order to realize that desire. There is sometimes a sexual motivation for being or looking like an amputee, called apotemnophilia, or a sexual attraction to people already missing limbs, called acrotomophilia. They can exist separately but most individuals exhibit both desires.

If I hold on for a while when I need to pee, will it give me better bladder control?

Some people have a particular type of incontinence called urge incontinence, which occurs when the need to pee comes on very suddenly, often before they can get to a toilet. It's most common in the elderly. One of the treatments for this is to learn to lengthen the time between urges to go to the bathroom. You'd start by urinating at set intervals, such as every 30 minutes to two hours (whether there is a need to go or not). This time is then gradually lengthened until you're urinating every three to four hours. This is essentially what you are asking, and so will help to discipline the bladder somewhat, although a healthy person with no continence issues probably does not need to do this.

Another form of bladder training involves stopping or slowing the urine flow midstream. The muscles that control this can then be identified and exercised on their own. These are known as Kegel exercises.

Did You Know... Women burn fat more slowly than men, by a rate of about 50 calories a day. Most men have a much easier time burning fat than women. Women, because of their reproductive role, generally require a higher basic body fat proportion than men, and as a result their bodies don't get rid of excess fat at the same rate as men.

I keep getting a smelly vaginal discharge even though I always douche my vagina regularly. What else can I do?

You can stop douching for a start. Douching is actually not necessary to keep the vagina clean and sweet smelling. It disrupts the body's natural protective cleansing system and rinses away the bacteria and yeast that are always present in the vagina and which stop other disease- and smell-causing bugs from growing. This is certainly what is happening to you. Your vagina should normally contain a lot of 'good' bacteria, called *lactobacilli*, which help keep the numbers of other bacteria, called *anaerobes*, down. Your regular douching is washing these lactobacilli away, allowing too many anaerobes to grow, which can cause a clear, fishy-smelling discharge.

Douching can also make it easier to catch STDs, bacterial and yeast infections, and HIV. The best thing to do is to leave your vagina alone and let your body's natural system work to keep it clean.

My periods are really heavy, with flooding and clots. I don't want to have a hysterectomy to stop them, but what else can be done?

Heavy periods can be extremely disabling, and if left can cause problems like anaemia.

There are many potential causes, such as hormonal imbalances, fibroids, polyps, infections and also problems with blood-clotting. Some women are more likely to have heavy bleeding than others, particularly those who are overweight, have never been pregnant, have thyroid problems or diabetes, and are over 35.

You will certainly need to use both a tampon and a sanitary towel during the first few days of your period, and may need to change the tampon every two hours.

It would be best to get your doctor to do some blood tests to check the balance of your hormones, as correcting these may well solve your problem.

You could try either taking the combined contraceptive pill or another medicine called tranexamic acid, which can shorten your periods. An anti-inflammatory medicine called mefenamic acid can also reduce the blood loss in heavy periods; there is a hormone tablet called norethisterone which could help, too.

When I laugh or sneeze I pee a bit. Also if I do certain exercise, like jogging, I leak urine. I tend to stay at home now because of this problem. What can I do?

This is most likely to be a condition called stress urinary incontinence, and is caused by a weakness of the urinary muscles, which are no longer able to hold your urine in under increased physical pressure, as when sneezing, coughing, laughing or during exercise.

There are loads of possible causes, but the most common is a prolapse. Fibroids and ovarian cysts can also be responsible. The main muscles that are weak are the bladder sphincter (the muscle that seals urine in the bladder), or what is known as 'detrusor instability' – weakness of the bladder muscle itself.

You really need to discuss this problem with your doctor, as there are a number of ways it can be successfully treated, including special exercises, physiotherapy, medication and surgery.

Is it possible to produce breast milk without being pregnant? I've recently come off the Pill and have some discharge coming from my nipples.

It *is* possible to produce breast milk when not pregnant. The hormone responsible for milk production is called prolactin and it is produced by the pituitary gland in the brain. Certain medications such as metoclopramide or thioridazine can cause your prolactin levels to rise and stimulate milk production. A rare cause of high prolactin levels is a benign growth in the pituitary gland that over-stimulates the prolactin-releasing tissue. Blood tests can be used to measure the level of hormones in your body, and an eye test can show whether or not there is any significant enlargement of the pituitary gland.

In older women, a condition called 'duct ectasia' can cause a milky discharge from the nipple. Most importantly, a discharge from the nipple can be a sign of a more sinister breast disease such as cancer, so you should always get it checked out by your doctor.

> **Did You Know...** Women's hair is about half the diameter of men's hair. While it might sound strange, it shouldn't come as too much of a surprise that men's hair should be coarser than that of women. Hair diameter also varies between races.

Does wearing antiperspirant deodorant really increase your chances of developing breast cancer?

There is no truth in this that has yet been revealed by extensive research. The theory was that by suppressing perspiration under the armpit, you prevent the excretion of toxins that then lead to breast cancer. This is biologically implausible, as your armpits are certainly not a route for 'toxin' excretion. They smell because of bacteria breaking down the sweat, not because of toxins.

Another theory suggested is that the aluminium salts in antiperspirants get absorbed into the body and block lymph glands around the breasts, eventually causing cancers. There is no evidence that this occurs, and no chemicals in deodorants have been found to be carcinogenic.

Are breast implants safe? There was so much stuff written about them in the papers at one time, but I'm not sure what the final conclusions were.

Initially the scares arose concerning the safety of silicone in breast implants. Silicone gel implants have now been extensively studied and, while there were initial concerns about their safety, which prompted wide professional debate and much media hype, the experts now regard those initial concerns as unfounded, and silicone is the more commonly used filler for implants.

Some implants are filled with saline, which is a natural substance within the body. Saline-filled implants can contract or deflate with time, but many come with a top-up valve in case this happens. Again, these are considered safe.

There were some implants produced called Trilucent, which contained soya-bean oil, which is translucent under X-ray. This would allow effective mammograms to be taken, if they were needed – something not easily done with other types of implant. It was subsequently found that if the implants ruptured and oil leaked into surrounding tissues, it caused swelling and inflammation that only settled when the implant was removed. They are now no longer used.

Can I increase the size of my bust without having implant surgery?

No, despite countless spam emails trying to convince you otherwise. Breasts do change in size under the influence of your hormones, and you might have noticed some changes at different times in your menstrual cycle, but that is as far as it goes. Pregnancy also makes a significant difference as the breasts prepare to produce milk, but these changes are only temporary. I have seen many adverts for exercises, creams, pills and 'secret techniques' for increasing your bust size, and none of them works. These products prey on the gullibility and psychological distress of people who wish to seek a change in their physical appearance, usually due to issues with self-esteem.

The best non-invasive way of increasing bust size is to use a push-up or padded bra, which at least gives the required appearance.

I am 16 and still haven't had my period. My friends all started theirs ages ago and now I feel that there must be something wrong with me. What can I do?

Not to have started your periods by the age of 16 is not so unusual. Everyone goes through the changes of puberty at his or her own speed. You should have noticed some changes occurring, however, like breast development and pubic hair growth. If you don't think anything has happened yet, then do go and see your doctor, who can test your hormone levels to check that everything is proceeding normally.

You could ask your mother at what age she started her periods. Many girls get their period at about the same age as their mothers did. So hereditary factors do play a part, but not exclusively. Being very underweight, eating disorders, or being extremely athletic can delay puberty and cause missed periods. I wouldn't worry unless you have noticed no changes to your body at all.

Did You Know... Your lips have a reddish colour because of the great concentration of tiny capillaries just below the skin. The blood in these capillaries is normally highly oxygenated and therefore quite red. This explains why the lips turn blue in very cold weather: cold causes the capillaries to constrict, so the blood loses oxygen and changes to a darker colour.

Is there such a thing as female ejaculation? I think I saw it in a porn film once but am not sure if it was made up.

This is still open to debate. Medical textbooks don't say much about it and we docs are certainly never taught anything on the subject, but there has been a recent upsurge of research into the female sexual response.

Many scientists now accept that some women can ejaculate some kind of fluid during sexual arousal or orgasm. Just how common it is, what the fluid is, and whether it serves any kind of function are hotly debated questions.

Less widely known is that women have prostate tissue, too. And this, it seems, is the best candidate for the source of female ejaculate. Also known as the Skene's glands or the para-urethral glands, they can produce a milky white prostatic fluid, similar to that formed in men. Women with large glands may well be the ones who can 'ejaculate'.

Why women should need to do this is a question rarely addressed. Some researchers have suggested that female ejaculation evolved to combat infections of the urethra and bladder. Many secretions and fluids produced by the human body, such as saliva, tears and, indeed, male ejaculate, are awash with compounds that inhibit the growth of bacteria. Urinary tract infections are relatively common in women, and sometimes arise from bacteria spread to the urethra during sex. A gush of antimicrobial fluid at the entrance to the urethra around the time of sex might help fight off such bacteria.

Why should girls wipe their bottoms from the back?

This is something that all little girls should be taught but often are not. It's all to do with urinary tract infections and trying to prevent them. UTIs are caused by bacteria entering the urethra and making their way up into the bladder, causing an infection.

Girls get urinary tract infections much more frequently than boys, almost certainly due to differences between the two sexes in the shape and length of the urethra. Girls have shorter urethras than boys, and the opening lies closer to the rectum and vagina, where bacteria are likely to be. These bugs can get into the urethra in several ways: during sex the bacteria in the vaginal area may be pushed into the urethra and eventually end up in the bladder, where urine provides a good environment for the bacteria to grow. Bacteria can also be introduced into a girl's bladder by wiping from back to front after a bowel movement, which can contaminate the urethral opening with faecal bacteria. This is why girls should wipe front to back after pooing, to avoid spreading bacteria from the rectal area to their urethra.

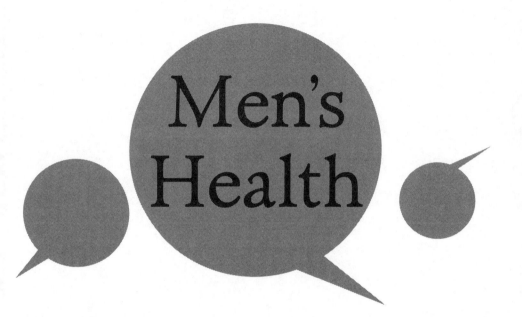

Men's
Health

When I was at school we always joked about getting 'scrot rot', but does it actually exist, and if so what is it?

It does indeed. Other charming terms for this condition include 'jock itch', 'Dhobi itch' or more simply, 'thrush'. The medical term is *Tinea cruris*. It tends to cause intense itching and soreness to the skin in your groin, and the area can become very red. A common fungal infection, it is usually caused by *Candida albicans* (thrush) or, as mentioned, Tinea.

Use any over-the-counter antifungal cream and keep the area cool and dry. Avoid synthetic pants or clothes as much as you can, as they make you sweat and exacerbate it. One top tip – if you have athlete's foot, you may be passing the infection from your feet to your groin as you put your pants on. Remember the phrase 'socks before jocks' and you won't do it again – put your socks on first, then your underwear.

What is gynaecomastia? Is it the same thing as moobs (man boobs) or not?

Man boobs and gynaecomastia are not, strictly speaking, the same thing, although the terms are often confused. Gynaecomastia is a common condition seen most often in teenage boys, where firm, tender breast tissue grows under the nipples, under the influence of hormones. It's usually caused by rising oestrogen levels during puberty, and will disappear without treatment within a couple of years. It's quite normal at that age. It can occur in adults taking anabolic steroids, certain medicines (prescription or over-the-counter) or using cannabis. Occasionally gynaecomastia may be due to a tumour or hormonal disease. You should consider having tests to find out the cause, as it can be linked to the pituitary gland, the liver or the testicles, and so treatment may be necessary. Options include medication to reduce the extra breast tissue or, in rare cases, surgery.

Moobs are not the same thing. They are, to put it bluntly, just fat, caused by poor diet, lifestyle and lack of exercise. This 'false gynaecomastia' does not involve any breast gland growth, and none can be felt when examined. They can be tackled by a good overhaul of lifestyle – drinking less and the introduction of a healthy eating plan and exercise.

Did You Know... The average life expectancy of a male born in the UK in 1997 is still less than 75 years. Men who are defined as 'partly skilled' or 'unskilled' have a life expectancy of less than 70 years. 41 per cent of all male deaths under the age of 75 (almost 60,000 a year in the UK) are caused by circulatory diseases, the largest single cause of death. Of these deaths, over two-thirds (some 41,000) are due to coronary heart disease. Each year, over 130,000 men of all ages die from circulatory diseases.

I'm a 19-year-old male and have a really high voice, which I hate. Is there anything that I can do to deepen it?

Your genetics dictates the way that you are, but there is always the possibility that you just might have fewer male hormones than some other men. It's probably best to let a doctor examine you to assess your body shape and hair distribution, and to check your genitalia and developmental stage. Any concerns and the doc can give you a blood test to measure some of your hormones or refer you to a specialist in glandular problems, known as an endocrinologist. Correcting this may help with your voice, but chances are you have developed quite normally. Cigarettes and whisky are probably not a wise choice of treatment. There are vocal coaches who may be able to teach you to lower your voice through certain exercises.

Can men get breast cancer if they don't have breasts?

Actually, yes they do and so yes they can, but it is rare. Out of all breast cancers, less than 0.5 per cent occur in men and it is very rare in men under 60, so men don't really need to check their breasts regularly.

The only known risk for male breast cancer is a chromosomal disorder called Klinefelter's syndrome. This seems to occur slightly more often in black men.

What is a normal penis size?

So many men worry about this, but there is no 'normal' or 'right-sized' penis, and everyone's is different. Some are huge, some are tiny, but according to research, the average penis size is about 8 cm (3.5 inches) when limp (flaccid), and about 13–15 cm (5–6 inches) when erect. There is a huge variation in floppy size, too, and the well-known phrase 'shower or grower' does have some truth behind it. Willies that look impressively large in the changing room probably won't get much bigger when erect, while penises that are smaller when limp expand more when erect. So limp size does not predict size when erect. Studies also show that very few men actually have longer than average penises when erect.

If you look at your penis from above, it will look smaller than it actually is. Your penis may also look smaller if you are overweight, as some of its base will be hidden by fat. Losing weight will make your penis appear larger, as will keeping pubic hair short. Remember that what you might have seen from watching porn will almost certainly be the exception to the rule, and not what most guys have!

How can I enlarge my penis? Do penis enlargement pills work?

Most men worry that their penis is too small, but many guys will actually have, in medical terms at least, an average-sized, and therefore normal, penis. Unfortunately the male ego is rarely happy to settle with 'average'. A penis would only be considered unusually small if it were less than 7.6 cm (3 inches) when erect. The vast majority of men who request a penis enlargement actually have a normal-sized penis.

There are two main surgical techniques for penis enlargement. The first increases the girth (width) of the penis by injecting fat taken from another part of the body, into the penis. Sometimes silicone is used instead of fat. It can result in an increase of around 4 cm (1.6 inches) to the girth.

The second technique is designed to increase the length of the penis. The ligament inside the penis is cut and stretched. The surgery usually results in an increase in length of around 2.5 cm (1 inch).

Both operations have complications like infection, loss of sensation, pain, incontinence and impotence.

As for enlargement pills, well, if they did work then, knowing the vanity of men, we would all sport monster willies, I suspect. They don't. There are many websites that offer so-called herbal penis enlargement pills or ointments. Despite the impressive claims made by these websites, there is absolutely no clinical evidence that these pills or ointments are effective.

More worrying is the fact that these unregulated herbal products could be dangerous for you. Analysis of some of the pills available on the internet found traces of lead, pesticides, the dangerous *E. coli* bacteria, and high levels of animal faeces. As so many women try to reassure their men: 'It's not the size of the boat, but the motion of the ocean that matters.'

Did You Know... 28 per cent of men still smoke. 27 per cent of men drink alcohol at a level that could be harmful to their health.

Is there any medical reason for so many men to have been circumcised? Is there any evidence that a circumcised penis is healthier than an uncircumcised one?

In a word: No. There is no reason for so many male babies to have been circumcised. Existing scientific evidence does demonstrate some potential medical benefits of being circumcised, like a reduced incidence of penile cancers, urinary tract infections (UTIs) and sexually transmitted diseases like HIV, but these benefits do not occur in large enough numbers to justify routinely circumcising all males. In fact, relying on circumcision to protect against these conditions is foolish and ill-advised.

Medical reasons for circumcising adults include an inability to retract the foreskin (phimosis), recurrent inflammation of the foreskin and the head of the penis (balanitis), and inflammation of the prepuce (posthitis). Complications of adult circumcision include a change in sensation during intercourse, bleeding, poor cosmetic results and infection.

I was circumcised as a baby and now have a very insensitive penis and hate the way it looks. Can I get my foreskin restored?

There is no real clinical reason to circumcise babies these days, and many men are unhappy that it was done. The great debate on whether circumcising is good or bad still rages, with arguments like loss of sensitivity, loss of protection, drying, callusing and aesthetic reasons being laid down by the anti-circumcision lobby, and those of greater hygiene, reduced incidence of HIV transmission and reduced rates of penile cancers on the pro side.

Foreskin-restoration techniques have been developed, but can take a long time to work. They often simply involve stretching the existing skin using little weights to pull it forward over the head of the penis. Clearly there is very little loose skin to start with, and since the skin cells only grow very slowly, just like skin growing over a graft or over an open wound, you can imagine it would take many months, even years, to achieve the growth of an artificial foreskin.

Have a look at the website www.norm-uk.org for more information on this subject.

I ripped my foreskin during sex. It is really sore and doesn't seem to be healing. What should I do?

You really need to see a urological surgeon to get it assessed. They can tell you whether it's necessary to do a surgical 'repair' on the foreskin – or whether you need a circumcision. Until then, take it very easy with sex and use lots of lubrication.

Is it true that you can actually break your penis?! I have heard stories of guys having over-enthusiastic sex and snapping it, but are these not just myths? A penis has no bones in, after all.

It *is* actually possible to fracture your penis. It doesn't have a bone in it but it does have a thick outer membrane that covers the erectile chambers, and this can get broken. It is not common but it can happen and is very painful when it does. It only occurs when you have an erection. It can happen when having sex or when wanking too forcefully. Guys who have experienced it often report hearing a popping or cracking sound when it happens, and the penis can turn a dark black/blue colour. It's considered a medical emergency and surgery is the best treatment for the injury. These days, the main aim of surgery would be to relieve the pain and prevent problems like erectile dysfunction, difficulty peeing and deformity. The faster the torn tissues can be repaired, the sooner the healing process can begin. Guys who fracture their willies are typically young, sexually active and highly motivated to resume sex as soon as they can. If it happens then I would strongly advise you to go to your GP and get a referral to a urologist to have it all assessed and, if necessary, repaired, or simply head straight for your nearest A&E.

Did You Know... The average man can expect to be seriously or chronically ill for 15 years of his life. The majority of men are too heavy for their health: 45 per cent are medically defined as overweight, and an additional 17 per cent as obese.

Why can't I use public toilets? I cannot urinate at a urinal if there are other men close to me.

It's surprisingly common for men to be unable to pee when other guys are around. It's not due to any physical cause, but is a sort of 'stage fright' and is known as *bashful bladder syndrome*. You may need to see a behavioural or cognitive psychotherapist, who could gradually accustom you to the idea of peeing near other people.

You can learn to 'decondition' yourself. You do this by, first, trying to pee in the cubicle of a public loo with the door shut. When you feel OK with this, you move on to having a pee with the door half open. Then you progress to peeing with the door fully open. Moving on from there, you select a very big public loo (for example, at a motorway service station) and practise peeing at a good distance from other guys. Over the next year, you can, in this way, gradually reduce the distance until you can cope with peeing quite near other folk.

Do men go through a drop in hormone levels like women do at the menopause?

Known by some as *andropause*, this is a rather controversial issue. It seems to be connected to the weariness, lack of motivation, lack of concentration and loss of sexual desire that many middle-aged men experience. There is no measurable fall in the levels of male hormones in the blood in mid-life (unlike in women, where the level of oestrogen falls dramatically at the menopause), but some researchers are convinced that, while the overall level of testosterone may not fall, the signalling molecules on the cells (which normally respond to testosterone) lose their sensitivity. This means that, although the hormone is there, the body isn't responding to it.

Hormone levels can be measured, and testosterone supplements are available on prescription in a variety of different forms including pills, patches and skin gels.

Replacing testosterone can improve a variety of conditions, including diabetes and erectile dysfunction.

Top 10 Health Threats to Men

1) Cancer

Lung cancer is the leading cause of cancer deaths among men, followed by prostate cancer and colorectal cancer. To reduce your risk of cancer never smoke, keep your weight within a healthy range by sticking to a careful diet and exercise regime, and drink only in moderation. Also limit your exposure to sunlight.

2) Heart Disease

The risk of contracting this threat to health can be reduced by making healthier lifestyle choices like not smoking, and eating a diet rich in vegetables, fruits, wholegrains, fibre and fish. Cut back on foods high in saturated fat and sodium. Treat any high blood pressure and raised cholesterol levels, and take regular exercise.

3) Injuries

The leading cause of fatal accidents for men is motor vehicle crashes, so always wear your seat belt, follow the speed limit, never drink or take drugs when driving and make sure you are well rested.

Falls and poisoning are other leading causes of fatal accidents. Placing carbon monoxide detectors near the bedrooms in your home can be lifesaving.

4) Stroke

You can't control all stroke risk factors, such as family history, age and race. But you can control others like smoking, high cholesterol and blood pressure.

5) COPD

Chronic obstructive pulmonary disease (COPD) is a group of chronic lung conditions, including bronchitis and emphysema. The main cause is often smoking, so again, don't!

6) Type 2 Diabetes

The most common type of diabetes, its complications include heart disease, blindness, and nerve and kidney damage. To prevent type 2 diabetes, lose weight if you are overweight, eat a diet rich in fruits, vegetables and low-fat foods, and include physical activity in your daily routine.

7) Flu

Influenza is a common viral infection the complications of which can be deadly, especially for those who have weak immune systems or chronic illnesses. Best thing you can do? Get a yearly flu jab.

8) Suicide

An important risk factor here is depression. If you feel you are depressed, consult your doctor, as treatment is available.

9) Kidney Disease

Kidney failure is often seen as a complication of diabetes or high blood pressure, so it is important you and your doctor keep these under control.

10) Alzheimer's Disease

There's no proven way to prevent Alzheimer's disease, but these steps may help: take care of your heart, avoid head injuries, keep your weight down, don't smoke and keep mentally fit.

I'm 21 but still do not grow stubble. I am small built and most people say I don't look my age. Is this normal?

There is huge variation in the amount of facial hair that men possess. Providing that you have gone through puberty, with normal sexual development and pubic hair, it's not an indication of any sort of hormonal problem. Some men, by nature, have very little beard growth, and not a great deal can be done about it. That is not to say that this won't change with time. It's not uncommon for facial hair to continue to increase in your late twenties and thirties. Mine did.

I occasionally have blood in my semen and it terrifies me. Is it serious?

Blood in semen can be very alarming to see, but is not usually serious and no treatment is needed. It is *not* caused by too much or too vigorous sex. It could be due to prostatic inflammation or even tiny stones in the bladder. Mild testicular irritation and possible sexual infections could cause it, too. It is rarely due to anything sinister like a cancer, but if it goes on then it is probably best to go for some tests to make sure all is well.

Did You Know... 31 per cent of all male deaths under the age of 75 (almost 48,000 a year in the UK) are caused by cancer, the second most common cause of death. Each year, over 124,000 men of all ages are newly diagnosed with cancer, and over 80,000 die. Prostate cancer is the most common cancer affecting men alone. Nearly 22,000 men in the UK are newly diagnosed with prostate cancer each year, and about 9,500 die. The number of new cases diagnosed is expected to treble over the next 20 years.

Every now and then I get a nasty red, blotchy irritation on the end of my penis. It can be itchy and quite uncomfortable. What could it be?

The most likely cause is a balanitis (an inflammation of the head of the penis, called the glans). It's not caught sexually but is due to an overgrowth of the normal organisms found under the foreskin. It is therefore more common in guys who have not been circumcised. It is important you retract and wash under your foreskin every day, and after sex. Treatment is not usually needed as it often settles down on its own, but some over-the-counter antifungal cream can help speed things up.

The best advice is to keep the area clean and dry. If you are getting recurrent thrush you need to be very persistent with treatments and continue any successful treatment for at least two weeks after the rash has disappeared, to prevent recurrence.

Occasionally, recurrent thrush can be a sign of early diabetes, so it may be wise to ask your GP if he or she would consider testing a specimen of your urine for glucose (sugar) levels.

Help! My penis is bending! Why is this happening?

Penises come in many shapes and sizes, particularly when limp. When they are erect they tend to be more similar in size and shape. A normal erect penis curves slightly, but can also go to one side by as much as 30 degrees without causing any problem.

If your penis seems to be curving more and more and is causing you pain, you may have a condition called Peyronie's disease. It affects 4 per cent of men over 40, and we don't know the exact cause, but it's thought to occur as the result of an injury to the penis when erect (which you may not have noticed). This causes the sponge-like erectile tissue to get inflamed, which can lead to scarring on the surface tissue of the penis. The inflammation and scarring causes the skin to toughen and contract, causing a

54

bend in the shaft of the penis. Some people might be genetically disposed to Peyronie's disease, as it can run in families.

Take a picture of your erect penis with a digital camera so you can show it to your GP to help with the diagnosis. It's very hard to diagnose Peyronie's from examining a flaccid penis: many urologists will induce an erection chemically in order to assess it properly.

Vitamin E supplements are sometimes effective in reducing pain and deformity. Medicines used to treat the condition include Tamoxifen, which is normally used to treat breast cancer, and Verapamil, which is often used to treat high blood pressure.

High-energy sound waves can also be used to reduce the pain and deformity.

Peyronie's disease of more than a year's standing which has not responded to other forms of treatment will probably need surgery to correct it.

One option involves cutting some tissue from the opposite side of the penis in order to balance out the affected area. The penis should then straighten, but it will be 1–3 cm (about 1 inch) shorter.

Another surgical technique is to implant some tissue, normally a vein from the groin or ankle, into the affected area. This makes the toughened area more flexible and there is no loss of penis size, however some men can have difficulties getting an erection after the operation.

Can you tell me a bit more about testicular cancer? Do you really just find a lump to know you have it? How can you reduce your risk?

Testicular cancer is the most common cancer among young men in the UK, but it's still rare and there are plenty of other causes of testicular lumps: epididymitis is an inflammation of the tubes that store sperm; scrotal cysts and hernias can give you lumps;

a hydrocoele is a collection of fluid in the scrotum and will feel like a soft lump; a varicocoele is a collection of distended blood vessels in the scrotum; epididymo-orchitis is an inflammation of the testicle often caused by a bacterial infection or a virus like mumps; the testicle can become twisted and will get swollen and painful.

You may notice pain and swelling in your testes or groin area, but actually only a small number of tumours are painful. A lump is the most common first sign, as is a feeling of heaviness in the scrotum. Sometimes a collection of fluid can occur in the scrotum, as can enlargement and tenderness of the breasts and general fatigue.

Risk factors include having undescended testicles: guys who have one testicle that never descended, even if it has been corrected surgically, are at greater risk. Age is another risk factor: testicular cancer affects younger men between the ages of 15 and 35 most commonly. It is also more common in white men.

Remember that the vast majority of testicular cancers are treatable and curable if caught early enough, so make sure you check your balls each month.

When I was younger I had a testicular cancer successfully treated, but want to know what effect this will have had on my fertility?

If you had the testicle removed, then this should not make any difference to your fertility provided that the other is working normally. Sometimes if the surgery was very disruptive and you had many lymph nodes removed, too, there may have been some damage to the nerves supplying erectile function and ejaculation, but you would have noticed this soon after the operation. If you had radiotherapy this can interfere with sperm production, but the effect would have only been temporary. Chemotherapy can affect fertility, which is why many men are now offered the chance to have sperm collected and frozen before treatment.

I have a rim of small spots all round the head of my penis. I am scared they might be warts, but I have had them for as long as I can remember. What should I do?

These sound like a totally harmless normal variation seen in a lot of guys called 'pearly penile papules', or more technically *hirsuties papillaris genitalis*. They are completely benign and not caused by a sexually transmitted infection. We are not sure why they form, but we do know they have nothing to do with sexual activity or personal hygiene. They are very common in men in their twenties and thirties, and uncircumcised men also report a high occurrence of these papules as well. If they are very prominent and unsightly and affect your confidence, they can be removed using carbon dioxide laser ablation, but this is rarely necessary.

Did You Know... Your brain operates on the same amount of power as 10-watt lightbulb. Your brain generates as much energy as a small lightbulb even when you're sleeping.

I am always reading about prostate cancer, but what exactly is your prostate? What does it do?

Your prostate is a small gland about the size of a walnut or small plum, which lies under your bladder just up inside your bottom. The tube through which you pee passes through the middle of it. Its job is to make the fluid that forms semen, the liquid that sperm swim in. It can develop chronic infections, can slowly enlarge affecting urinary function, and can also develop cancers. Symptoms of these problems include pain, an increased urge to pee, difficulty peeing, dribbling after peeing and having to get up frequently in the night to pee. A very common condition which a lot of men get in their prostate from the age of about 50 is benign prostatic hypertrophy, or BPH. It has nothing to do with cancer but it can obstruct urine flow, causing the symptoms described above. Treatments include doing nothing if the symptoms are not too bothersome, taking medications to shrink the gland, and surgery to reduce the constriction of the urethra.

Does your penis really shrink as you get older? Old men I have seen do seem to have much smaller willies than younger guys.

No, they don't, you will be relieved to hear. Otherwise there really isn't much to look forward to in old age, is there? Actually your penis size remains much the same from puberty onwards, but the amount of abdominal and pubic fat increases, burying your penis and making it appear smaller. The strength and frequency of erections does decrease, however. Keeping your weight down as you age will help you avoid the 'shrinking penis' problem.

The piece of skin connecting my foreskin to my penis broke, causing pain and bleeding. Does it need reconnecting?

This is colloquially known as 'snapping the banjo string' and can sometimes occur if you have a rather short join between the area just in front of the head of your penis and the foreskin. The small piece of skin in question is called the *frenulum*, which you have broken. It may right itself over two weeks or so if left, although sometimes scarring may occur, leading to a shorter frenulum than before and recurrent problems. If so, then an adult circumcision would be the best solution, so I suggest you go to see your doctor for advice.

Why is it that when I lie still I can see my balls moving around? They do it in the bath and when I am warm in bed. Is it normal?

All men know that their testicles hang loose when it's warm and retract up into their bodies in cold weather. They do the same thing if they come into contact with cold water. They hang in a bag of skin called the scrotum and are anatomically positioned 'outside' the body to keep them below normal body temperature. This makes them biochemically more efficient at carrying out their two main functions – making sperm and making and releasing testosterone – but it also makes them rather vulnerable, as every boy knows.

There exists, therefore, an interesting if somewhat defunct reflex called the *cremasteric reflex*. If you stroke the upper inner part of your thigh, your testicles will move away from the side being touched. This reflex evolved to help keep the testicles out of harm's way when we used to walk about naked.

Two main muscles are involved in the movements that you can see: the cremaster, described above, and the dartos muscle, which helps move the testicles up and down inside the scrotum.

The main reason you see them move relates to temperature regulation. The cremaster muscle expands and contracts according to temperature.

Interestingly, your testicles also move during sexual arousal. They elevate just before ejaculation to make direct contact with the body, and they increase in size due to vasocongestion, the accumulation of blood in the pelvis that occurs during arousal.

If sexual excitement is sustained long enough, the testicles can almost double in size, returning to normal size after orgasm. So yes, the movements you can see are normal.

Did You Know... The strongest muscle in the human body is the tongue. While you may not be able to lift much with it, it is in fact the strongest muscle relative to its size.

I have a large varicose vein in one testicle. Should it be treated and if so how?

Varicosed scrotal veins, known as a varicocoele, are often associated with a dull ache, especially on standing. In some men a large varicocoele can interfere with erectile function. Because they bring an increased blood flow to the area they can raise the temperature of the testicles and so reduce sperm quality and quantity. All this means that if the symptoms are thought to be significant, if the size of the veins give cause for concern, or if there are fertility issues, then you can have it removed surgically. If not, then you may simply leave it alone. The operation involves an incision being made in the scrotum and then the abnormal veins are cut and tied, and the tortuous dilated vein removed. Recovery is usually complete within one week.

Did You Know... The suicide rate among men is increasing. The rate has doubled among 15- to 24-year-old men in the past 25 years.

I love to cycle but my friends tease me that it will make my penis shrink – can this really be true?

Unfortunately there is actually some truth in this jibe. The very action and pressures of cycling can put too much pressure on the perineum, causing the penis and scrotum to contract. It's known among sportspeople as 'gym balls' or 'saddle balls'.

I note your friends didn't mention impotence to you. Although the jury's still out on the subject of whether bicycle riding causes 'cycling impotence' – largely because there has been no qualified or scientifically acceptable studies carried out on the subject – there is plenty of anecdotal and clinical evidence to confirm that long-term or endurance cycling causes numbness and discomfort in the genital region, as well as temporary impotence.

Part of the problem lies in the fact that the long, narrow and hard saddle shape pushes into the perineum and compresses the nerves and major blood vessels that supply the penis and ultimately control and maintain an erection.

The number of teenage bike riders consulting doctors about impotence problems has certainly increased, most likely due to blunt trauma injuries that occur when performing cycling stunts like jumps and going down steps.

One urologist colleague of mine says that there are two kinds of cyclists: those who are impotent and those who will be.

It can be avoided by investing in a good, anatomically correct saddle.

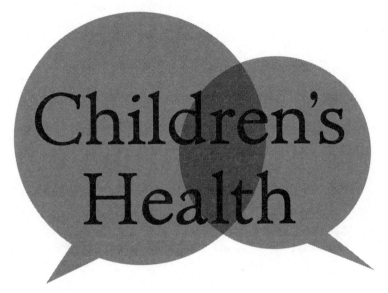

Is it true that sugar makes kids hyperactive?

The classic situation is after a children's party: wild, out-of-control youngsters tearing around the house, overloaded with excitement and seemingly high on the sugary party food. But it's not actually the sugar that's to blame.

Loads of studies have been done that show that sugar does not affect children's behaviour – though most parents, understandably, find this hard to believe. An analysis of the available data looked at 12 large-scale studies, some of which looked specifically at children with attention deficit hyperactivity disorder (ADHD), and no differences in behaviour were found between children who had had sugar and those who had not. An article published in the *Journal of Abnormal Child Psychology* reported on research that showed that the supposed increase in hyperactive behaviour is actually more likely to come from parents' expectations. In the study, parents were told that their kids had been given sugar, and were then asked to rate their children's behaviour. The adults reported a far higher rate of behavioural problems in their children for the next few hours – but the truth was their kids had only been given a sugar-free juice drink. This shows that parents who think that their child has consumed a sugary drink will label the child's behaviour as hyperactive, even if the child has actually not consumed any sugar.

The assumption that sugar causes hyperactivity is almost certainly due to something that researchers call a 'confounding' factor. Sugary foods and drinks are usually laced with other substances such as food colourings, flavourings, preservatives and sweeteners. The evidence suggests that it is much more likely to be these that are affecting children's behaviour. Sugar is the confounding factor, as although it is also present, it is not actually responsible for the behavioural changes.

Is it bad to let our dog lick my children's faces? My mother says it will make my kids blind and now I feel terrible!

Letting a dog lick your children's faces will probably not harm them. Obviously it's not the most hygienic thing to do, as dogs do sniff other dogs' faecal matter and eat some pretty revolting things. Well, mine certainly does! A common bug that you might get from kissing your dog is a streptococcal throat infection, which has been reported as being more prevalent among families who have dogs and children who kiss them.

Another possible risk, and the one that your mother is probably referring to, is that of catching roundworms (*Toxocara canis*), which can cause blindness. Although the risk is very small, humans can become infected with the worms by ingestion of eggs from soil contaminated by dog faeces. The appeal that puppies have to young children, and the great love small children have for putting things in their mouths, puts them at particular risk, but direct contact with dogs is not normally a route of transmission.

Did You Know... Child survival rates differ significantly around the world – three-quarters of child deaths occur in Africa and South-East Asia. About two-thirds of these deaths are preventable through access to practical, low-cost interventions, and effective primary care up to five years of age.

My two-year-old son has an awful habit of holding his breath when he is upset or has tantrums. He can turn blue and become unconscious, and it terrifies me. How can I prevent it and what do I do if it happens again?

Your son is having typical breath-holding attacks, which are quite common in young children but nevertheless can be really frightening for parents. There are two types: the 'blue' type where the child empties his lungs, stops breathing, goes blue and faints (which your son seems to experience), and the more rare 'pale' or 'faint' type which can happen after a painful or frightening experience. Neither type will harm your child in any way, and children usually grow out of them, often by the time they reach school age. In the meantime, when he does it all you need do is protect him from hurting himself if he falls to the floor. Blowing in his face, as some parental guides suggest, is really not necessary, as he will breathe again by himself.

What's the best way to feed a toddler?

From around six months of age you can start to give your baby some solid foods. As she grows, start to introduce more textures and tastes by feeding purées and crunchy raw carrots, and then move on to small pieces of food that will need to be chewed. It's important that you make sure her diet contains a balance of vitamins and minerals from all the food groups, as she is growing quickly. Meat, fish, dairy products, dried fruit, green vegetables and pulses are all excellent sources of iron and protein. Full-fat milk and dairy foods provide calcium for strong bones and teeth, bread and cereals provide lots of energy, and five small portions of fruit and vegetables a day will give plenty of fibre. I would suggest that you avoid anything containing raw eggs or raw shellfish, which can cause serious food poisoning. Nuts should be crushed or flaked, as whole ones could cause choking, but avoid if there is a strong family history of nut allergy. It's better to offer a variety of nutritious snacks and smaller meals than trying to feed her large meals in one go.

How do I know if my child is being abused?

This is something no one wants to have to think about but is important to know in order to prevent it happening. Abuse can be classified into four types: physical, sexual, emotional, and neglect. More than one of these may be suffered at the same time.

It can be very difficult to be absolutely sure if abuse really is occurring, and it is crucial to remember that an accusation of abuse can have devastating consequences, but there are certain signs that may indicate it is happening. Unexplained cuts, bruises, burns, bite or welt marks on a child's body, and/or soreness, pain or bruises around the genitals or mouth are all possible clues, as are changes in the child's behaviour. This may include becoming withdrawn, secretive or very clingy, fearing adults, developing problems in school, having nightmares, bedwetting, and showing aggressive or anti-social behaviour. If the abuse is of a sexual nature, then the child may show an inappropriate interest in or knowledge of sexual acts, out of proportion for his age. Conversely, he may avoid talking about anything related to sexuality and sex altogether.

Please remember that any of these signs may have a variety of other explanations and does not necessarily mean that a child is being abused – bedwetting is a common condition that can affect any child, for instance, so use your common sense, but don't be afraid to speak up if you're worried about any child.

Did You Know... Between 3 and 8 per cent of the babies born each year will be affected by developmental disorders such as attention deficit hyperactivity disorder or mental retardation.

When should I begin to talk to my kids about sex?

Many people find talking about sex difficult and embarrassing, but you mustn't let this stop you giving your child a good education about the facts of life. Most people in my medical speciality would agree that teaching sexuality to children is probably more important than teaching them table manners or how to do up their shoes! Being aware of his or her body and sex from an early age will mean that your child will understand right from wrong and, importantly, will be able to identify if an adult behaves or touches inappropriately. Showing that it is OK to talk openly about sex will let your children know they can always come to you if they have any worries, and discussing issues such as pregnancy and sexually transmitted infections with older children will help to normalize these issues and make them less taboo. It will also teach them to take precautions and look after themselves.

It is a total myth that educating your children about sex will encourage them to go out and start doing it. In fact, knowing the facts and issues often makes children less likely to experiment before they are ready. The key is to allow them to make up their own minds when it comes to sex, and not be pressured into anything they don't want to do.

I suggest you start from an early age, as this will make it less awkward for both you and your child. Puberty can be a scary time for children, so explain to them what is happening to their bodies and why. Sex education should be a gradual progression from a young age, not a toe-curlingly embarrassing one-off lecture when children reach their teens.

And remember, sex is not just purely a physical or mechanical process. Talk about the emotional aspects of making love, too. Don't let sex become a taboo subject, as a child could grow up believing sex is wrong, when in fact it is part of a normal, healthy relationship between humans.

Did You Know... Pneumonia is the largest single cause of death in children under five years of age. Out of 154 million cases each year, nearly three-quarters occur in just 15 countries.

How can I tell if my child has ADHD?

Attention deficit hyperactivity disorder (ADHD) is the most common behavioural disorder that starts in childhood. In the UK it affects around 5 per cent of children. It's a medical condition that should not be confused with normal excitable, or boisterous, childhood behaviour. It can run in families and it's thought that the condition is caused by an imbalance of certain chemicals in the brain. As a result of the imbalance, the brain has difficulty processing all the information and stimulants that it receives.

The symptoms of ADHD usually start around the age of four. The classic signs include poor concentration, being easily distracted, restlessness, fidgety behaviour, difficulty sitting down or remaining still when told to, difficulty following instructions, difficulty waiting one's turn in a group situation, and interrupting others. Affected children also have difficulty playing quietly, often shifting from one incomplete activity to another, and they may have little or no sense of danger, making them take part in potentially hazardous activities without thinking about the consequences. Different children with ADHD will have different symptoms.

There is no cure for ADHD, but treatment is available that can help you to cope with the emotional aspects of the condition and to control its symptoms.

Top 10 Culturally-bound Disorders

1) Koro

A psychological disorder characterized by delusions of penis shrinkage and retraction into the body, accompanied by panic and fear of dying. This delusion is rooted in Chinese metaphysics and cultural practices. Koro was thought to be transmitted through food. In 1967 there was a Koro epidemic in Singapore after newspapers reported cases of Koro due to eating pork which came from a pig that had been inoculated against swine fever. Not only did pork sales go down, but hundreds of Koro cases followed. This was more likely caused by mass hysteria.

2) Shenkui

A Chinese culture-bound syndrome involving marked anxiety or panic symptoms with accompanying physical complaints for which no physical cause can be found. Symptoms include dizziness, backache, fatigue, weakness, insomnia, frequent dreams and complaints of sexual dysfunction. Symptoms are attributed to excessive semen loss from frequent intercourse, masturbation, nocturnal emission, or passing of 'white turbid urine' believed to contain semen. Excessive semen loss is feared in some Chinese cultures because it represents the loss of one's vital essence and is therefore thought to be life threatening.

3) Gururumba

This disorder is specific to New Guinea and means a 'wild man' episode in which the sufferer (typically a married male) begins by burglarizing neighbouring homes, taking objects that he thinks are valuable but which seldom are. He may then run into a nearby forest, returning a number of days later without the objects and with amnesia. Sufferers appear hyperactive and clumsy with slurred speech.

71

4) Saora Disorder

Seen among the Saora tribe of Orissa State in India, this is characterized by young men and women exhibiting abnormal behaviour patterns that Western trained mental health specialists would likely define as a mental disorder. They may cry and laugh at inappropriate times, have memory loss, pass out and claim to experience the sensation of being repeatedly bitten by ants when no ants are present. Those affected are usually teenagers or young adults under considerable psychological stress from social pressure placed on them by their relatives and friends.

5) Berserkers

This term is recorded in old Norse literature and used to describe the fury affecting men and known as *berserkergang*, which occurred not only in the heat of battle, but also during laborious work. Affected men performed feats which did not normally seem humanly possible. This condition is said to have begun with shivering and chattering of the teeth, which led to a great rage, where those affected would howl like wild animals, bite the edge of their shields and cut down everything they met without discriminating between friend or foe.

6) Wendigo Psychosis

A mental disorder that affected Native Americans of the Algonquian-speaking tribes in which sufferers intensely crave human flesh and think they are turning into cannibals. Wendigo sufferers may threaten those around them or act violently or anti-socially. While some have denied the existence of this disorder, there are a number of credible eyewitness accounts that strongly suggest that Wendigo psychosis is a real phenomenon.

7) Ghost Sickness

Afflicting some Native American tribes and believed to be caused by association with the dead or dying, this is sometimes associated with witchcraft. It is considered to be a psychotic disorder of Navajo origin causing symptoms of general weakness, loss of appetite, a feeling of suffocation, recurring nightmares and a pervasive feeling of terror. The sickness is attributed by sufferers to ghosts (*chindi*).

8) Homosexual Panic

A term first coined by psychiatrist Edward J Kempf in 1920, describing an acute, brief reactive psychosis involving delusions and hallucinations that accuse the sufferer of various homosexual activities. The condition most often occurs in people who suffer schizoid personality disorders. Breakdowns often occur in situations that involve enforced intimacy, like dormitories or military barracks, and indeed it was most common during the mass mobilization of the Second World War when barracks typically provided little privacy. The condition may lead to suicidal or homicidal acts.

9) Couvade Syndrome

A condition which involves a father experiencing some of the behaviour of his wife at or near the time of childbirth, including her birth pains, postpartum seclusion, food restrictions and sex taboos. The term originally referred to the medieval Basque custom in which the father, during or immediately after the birth of a child, took to bed, complained of having labour pains and was accorded the treatment usually shown women during pregnancy or after childbirth. In some extreme cases, fathers can grow a belly similar to that of a 7-month pregnant woman and gain considerable weight.

10) Grisi Siknis

Translated as 'crazy sickness', this is a contagious, culture-bound syndrome that occurs among the Miskito People of Eastern Central America and affects mainly young women. During the attack, the victim loses consciousness of herself and views other people as devils. Some grab machetes or broken bottles to ward off unseen assailants. Other victims are reported to have performed superhuman feats, vomited strange objects such as spiders, hair and coins, and spoken in tongues. They feel no pain from injuries and have absolute amnesia regarding their physical circumstances.

What painkillers can I give my children?

Babies aged between two and three months old, as long as they weigh over 4 kg (8.8 lb), can be given children's liquid paracetamol for fever or discomfort. They can have up to two doses, four to six hours apart, but if the fever doesn't get better, or if your baby is ill for any other reason, it's important to seek medical advice. Children and babies over three months old can be given liquid paracetamol, and older children can take tablets, or tablets dissolved in water.

Children and babies over three months old can also have ibuprofen as long as they weigh over 5 kg (11 lb) and they don't have a history of asthma, heart problems, kidney problems, stomach ulcers or indigestion. Don't give your child ibuprofen if he has a history of any previous adverse reactions or sensitivity to it.

Never give aspirin to children under 16 years of age, as it can cause Reye's syndrome, a potentially fatal disease that causes numerous detrimental effects to many organs, especially the brain and liver. Pregnant women should avoid taking aspirin for the same reason.

Did You Know... A child's risk of dying is highest in the first month of life, when safe childbirth and effective neonatal care are essential. Preterm birth, birth asphyxia and infections cause most newborn deaths.

I'm 14 and it's taking forever for my voice to break. I squeak when I speak and it sounds terrible. Everything else seems to be developing normally apart from this. How long will it take?

This is a great question, but sadly there's no definitive answer. It might take weeks, months, or even a couple of years. The only important thing is maybe to check that there is no underlying problem with your hormones, but as you say all else is well then this sounds unlikely.

The changes in your voice are due to the thickening effects of the testosterone working on the tissues around your voice box. Don't change anything you are doing, and, as you've had six months of this already, I suspect it'll settle down pretty soon now. Many boys spend a period of time squeaking and growling away until their voices settle down into their adult pitch.

My son has to go into hospital to have an operation for hypospadias. What exactly is this condition, and is the operation successful and safe?

Hypospadias is a developmental abnormality of the urethra and penis that is present at birth. The main problem is that the urethra opens on the underside of the penis instead of at the end of the penis; this can be anywhere from just below the normal position (mild) to as far back as the base of the scrotum (severe). It can cause problems when peeing and also with erections in adults.

It's not a genetic condition but it can run in families, and around 1 in 300 boys is born with some degree of hypospadias. Reports suggest that it is becoming more common, but the reason why it occurs is not known.

If the abnormality is very slight then it can be left, but cases usually need to be corrected surgically. The extent of the surgery depends on the exact degree of hypospadias, but will involve the surgeon moving the exit of the urethra to a more normal position. It is a common operation and has a good outcome.

Will thumb-sucking ruin my baby's teeth?

Tired, stressed out and sleep-deprived parents may well feel grateful for a thumb-sucking habit as it stops the baby from crying and gives the parents some peace. Indeed thumb-sucking, or giving the baby a dummy, used to be encouraged. Then concerns were raised about the effect this was having on developing teeth. Investigators have found that there are two important factors that may influence whether thumb-sucking will cause teeth to stick out: the age at which it occurs, and the intensity, or strength, and frequency of sucking. Most dentists would agree that it won't harm baby teeth, but it shouldn't be allowed to continue once the permanent teeth arrive, usually around the age of six. If sucking displaces the emerging adult teeth then they will certainly need the attention of an orthodontist. Thumb- or finger-sucking can cause abnormal alignment of teeth, known as a malocclusion (the classic 'buck-toothed' appearance), and can also damage the roof of the mouth. These sorts of deformities can cause speech problems, such as a lisp.

As with all aspects of child (and animal!) training, positive reinforcement is always preferable to negative comments and punishments, which may only increase the problem by increasing the child's anxiety. Reward your child when he doesn't suck his thumb, rather than scolding him when he does.

Remember that sucking is a habit, and to be successful children will actually have to *want* to quit. As with most habits it will take about 30 to 60 days to let go of the urge to suck.

Why do some children get warts?

Warts are caused by the human papilloma virus, of which there are over 100 different types. The virus loves warm, moist places, and easily enters small cuts and scratches on the hands or feet, which is certainly one reason why children get them often. About 25 per cent of the population are susceptible to the human papilloma virus. The rest of us are immune to it, and never grow any warts. The virus is widespread in the community and cannot be avoided. When the virus enters through our skin, it replicates extremely slowly until it induces the growth of a wart at that site. Warts can grow for many months, or even a year or more, before they are big enough to be seen. Eventually the body develops antibodies to the wart virus, which cause the wart to drop off and give us protection against further warts developing. Children who bite their fingernails get warts more often than those who don't, but doctors really don't know why some kids get warts and others don't. Some people are just more likely to catch the wart virus than others, just as some people catch colds easily. Patients with a weakened immune system also are more prone to a wart virus infection.

Did You Know... Diarrhoeal diseases are a leading cause of sickness and death among children in developing countries. Exclusive breastfeeding helps prevent diarrhoea among young children. Treatment of sick children with oral rehydration salts has saved the lives of more than 50 million children in the last 25 years.

I am really worried about all the risks associated with vaccines, and don't want my children to have any. I hear that homoeopathic vaccines are just as effective and want to know if they are a suitable alternative.

Let's get one thing straight here: no form of homoeopathic treatment works any better than a placebo (nothing at all). And when it comes to vaccines, homoeopathic ones are downright dangerous, as they offer your child no protection whatsoever against the potentially life-threatening childhood diseases polio, diphtheria and whooping cough.

It is vital that as many children as possible have proper conventional vaccines, as an epidemic could arise if the vaccination rate among all children drops too low. Children given homoeopathic vaccines have gone on to develop the diseases the treatment was supposed to prevent, and this has resulted in death, disablement and permanent damage to hundreds of children.

Measles and mumps are often mild diseases, but in a significant proportion of children they can cause severe illness and, in a few children, permanent brain damage or even death.

Homoeopathic remedies have no proven record of success, and have been discounted by every reputable scientist. The risks of conventional vaccinations are infinitesimal, and far less than the risk associated with catching any of these diseases.

How do I tell if my child is ready to start toilet training, and what's the best way to go about it?

The two biggest mistakes parents make when it comes to toilet training are starting too early and putting too much pressure on the child. It has sometimes been said of potty training that the earlier you start, the later you'll finish.

Pressuring children can lead to power struggles, as well as a lot of angst and frustration on both sides. Children can also become constipated if they're under too much pressure, and get stressed or upset about using the toilet.

You really just need to let your child take the lead. Most children are physically and psychologically ready from around two-and-a-half years old, but it really depends on the child. Clues that he is ready include showing an interest when you use the bathroom, remaining dry for longer periods of time, or after a nap, and being aware of the fact he's about to go and knowing how to 'hold' it. Being bothered by a wet or dirty nappy is a clue, too.

The best way is to start gently by letting him watch you in the bathroom and explaining the process to him. Buy a potty or children's toilet seat and just have it around. Let your child simply sit on the toilet or potty, clothed or otherwise, for a minute or two before bathtime to help make it just another part of the routine. Teach your child in stages. Learning to pull his pants up and down, or to wash his hands on his own, are all individual stages. With all aspects of behavioural training, always praise success, and don't punish failure. Remember that accidents happen, often simply because a child is too busy playing and doesn't notice he needs to go until it's too late.

Be patient. Like every other skill your child has mastered, toilet training will take time and he's doing the best he can. Just stay positive and supportive and eventually he will be successful.

Did You Know... Leukaemia is the most common cancer in children under 15, accounting for 30 per cent of all childhood cancers, followed by brain and other nervous system cancers. In the West, cancer is the second leading cause of death among children aged 1 to 14 years of age, with unintentional injuries being the leading cause.

I have been told my son has dyspraxia. I don't really understand what this means or what to do. Can you explain? I read that evening primrose oil may help – should I try it?

Dyspraxia is becoming more widely recognized and is thought to affect around 2 per cent of the population. It's more common in boys. It is a developmental problem in which messages from an immature or underdeveloped brain are not properly transmitted to the rest of the body. It can affect multiple areas of development including intellectual, emotional, physical, language, social and sensory, and it can cause learning difficulties. People with dyspraxia often have a poor understanding of the messages their senses convey, and so have difficulty turning those messages into actions. Toddlers may be slow to feed themselves or in learning to dress, and young children can seem clumsy and lacking in co-ordination. It can often lead to bullying and problems at school as they get older. Poor handwriting is one of the most common symptoms, but is obviously very non-specific.

Any brain injury can result in dyspraxia, either by cells not developing properly in the womb, or from a lack of oxygen during birth. It can also follow brain damage caused by illness, stroke or an accident later in life. There is no cure, but those affected can learn ways to get around their difficulties and can lead normal lives. Involvement of occupational therapists, speech and language therapists, psychologists and specialist teachers may be needed during childhood, depending on the various ways that the child is affected.

Evening primrose oil and also cod liver oil contain essential fatty acids that are important for brain and neurological development. If you stick to the recommended doses it certainly won't do any harm, but there is no firm evidence for their effectiveness as yet.

My two-year-old son is talking much less than his sister did at 18 months. I heard that boys can start speaking later than girls, but should I be worried? When should he start to speak more?

By the age of two many children are babbling away incessantly, and should be joining two or three words together. It is perfectly normal for some children to do this later than others, but studies have shown that most catch up normally in the end.

It's a commonly told tale that boys talk later than girls, but as there is a huge variation in what is a 'normal' timeframe anyway, it makes showing a clear difference between the sexes hard to prove.

One thing I would advise is that you get his hearing assessed by his GP, as this is a common cause of late talking. If he is playing and interacting normally then it is unlikely there is any developmental problem or autistic condition, but if you are worried then these can be checked for, too.

Did You Know... From one month up until the age of five years, the main causes of loss of life are pneumonia, diarrhoea, malaria, measles and HIV. Malnutrition still contributes to more than half of all child deaths worldwide.

Can you tell me about artificial food colourings and what they do to children?

There is still much controversy over these additives. In the US, the Food & Drug Administration says that they are safe, but some groups in the US, like the Center for Science in the Public Interest, insist that they are not and want them banned. A study was published by Southampton University in 2007 that suggested a link between certain mixtures of food colours and the preservative sodium benzoate with hyperactivity in children, but opinions published in November 2009 concluded that the currently available data, including the Southampton University study, were not enough to prove a link between these individual colours and possible behavioural effects. It still prompted the European Food Safety Authority (EFSA) to begin re-evaluating the safety of all permitted food colourings, however, and now several new studies have become available. Already the use of the red colouring Red 2G has been restricted, and the rest of the re-evaluations of all food colours is expected to be completed in the middle of 2011. Until then it may be best to keep consumption of these to a minimum.

If you are concerned about any additives then remember that, by law, food additives must be listed on the label of the food in question, making them easier for you to avoid.

My son was shown how to change his voice by inhaling helium from party balloons, and now likes to do it as often as he can. I'm worried that it may be bad for him. What are the risks?

Loads of children (and quite a few adults, too) enjoy the resulting squeaky high-pitched change that temporarily happens to their voice when helium is inhaled. Generally speaking, this is quite harmless. Neutral helium at standard conditions is non-toxic, plays no biological role, and is found in trace amounts in human blood.

I think it would only be dangerous if done to excess, because the helium may displace oxygen needed for normal respiration. Helium gas in the lungs will create a diffusion gradient that washes out the oxygen, so that each breath of helium you take draws more oxygen out of your system. Helium does not provide any nourishment to the organs or the brain, and so, as the brain can only manage being deprived of oxygen for a very short time before unconsciousness occurs, if really enormous breaths of helium were taken then it's possible it might cause collapse.

One protecting factor is that our breathing reflex is not triggered by insufficient oxygen, but by an excess of carbon dioxide, and so no long-term harm would result.

This is all presuming that the helium is being inhaled from an inflated balloon. If it is inhaled directly from pressurized gas cylinders, then the high flow rate could fatally rupture lung tissue.

Of course you would be putting yourself in real danger if you climbed inside a giant helium balloon, as two college students did in Florida. They died.

It's little known that doctors actually use a mixture of helium and oxygen (called 'heliox') to help patients with upper-respiratory blockages. It works because the helium is a very light gas, and can more easily be pushed through an obstructed airway.

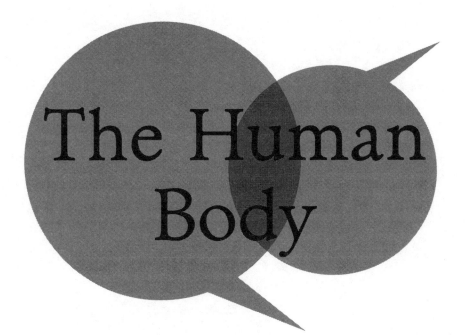

The Human Body

Why do we never forget how to ride a bike, and yet often can't remember names of old school friends or phone numbers?

When you first learned to ride a bike you were learning a motor skill, co-ordinated by the part of your brain called the cerebellum. There is a particular type of nerve cell called a *molecular layer interneuron* that encodes signals leaving the cerebellum so they can be stored as memories in other parts of the brain. So the muscle memory of riding a bike is stored very widely across the brain, unlike names and phone numbers. It's almost certainly an evolutionary mechanism that evolved to preserve important skills in case of injury.

How much memory does our brain have?

A human brain cell can hold five times as much information as the *Encyclopaedia Britannica*, or any other encyclopaedia for that matter. Scientists have yet to settle on a definitive amount, but the storage capacity of the brain in electronic terms has been estimated to be from 3 to as much as 1,000 terabytes. The National Archives in Britain, containing over 900 years of history, takes up only 70 terabytes, making your brain's memory power rather impressive indeed.

Do those 'brain-training' games actually work to improve your mental agility?

The market is swamped with games claiming to boost brain power and mental agility. But many studies have been done into the effects of brain exercises and the results have been mixed. One found that six weeks of computer brain training has little benefit beyond boosting performance on the specific tasks included in the training. The conclusion was that the results could not produce any evidence for any overall improvements in cognitive function following brain training. Another investigation by the consumer charity *Which?* concluded that 'none of the claims of commercial brain-training products are supported by peer-reviewed research published in a recognised scientific journal.' But some neuroscientists think otherwise. While they may agree that many of the brain-training products on the market are probably ineffective, they still think that cognitive functions can be trained, and that specific training paradigms can be effective. My advice? A healthy diet, exercise and a good book should be just as good for you.

Did You Know... The human heart creates enough pressure to squirt blood 30 feet.

Why do we hiccup? And especially, why do we hiccup when we are drunk?

The truth is that we don't know exactly why we get hiccups, but it is a universal phenomenon. Even foetuses in the womb can be seen and felt to hiccup on occasion, especially during the last trimester of pregnancy.

There is a correct medical term for hiccups: *singultus* (from a Latin word that describes the catching of the breath while crying). They involve a complex reflex of a sudden contraction of the diaphragm and the muscles between the ribs, causing air to be inhaled. This contraction ends almost as soon as it starts with 'glottic closure': the space in the throat near the vocal cords snaps shut, producing the typical sound. What you may not know is that, in most cases, only one of the two sides of the diaphragm is involved; in 80 per cent of cases, the left.

Hiccups have a number of triggers including emotional stress or excitement, overeating, drinking fizzy drinks, and smoking.

While they are usually an entirely benign experience, prolonged hiccups may be a sign of disease. Then the cause is usually irritation of one of the nerves in the chest, either by laryngitis, goiters (enlargement of the thyroid gland), tumours in the neck, infections near the diaphragm, or hiatus hernias. Rarer causes are aortic aneurysms and multiple sclerosis. Contrary to popular belief, alcohol does not significantly increase the occurrence of hiccups, but when they do occur while drinking they can last longer due to the nerve signal-depressing effects of alcohol. Traditional cures include dropping a cold key down one's back, getting a fright or drinking a glass of water backwards. They are all designed to distract the hiccup sufferer from his plight, allowing the muscle spasms to settle.

Why do we yawn, and why is yawning so contagious?

All vertebrate animals yawn, several times a day by some estimates, more often in the early morning and late evening. A foetus in the womb yawns as early as week 11 of development. Yawning does not always indicate that you are tired: it's true that people often yawn before going to bed, but they also yawn in the morning and at other times during the day, depending on a variety of factors like arousal level, distraction and, as everyone has experienced, seeing someone else yawning.

Some theories explain yawning as a reflex in response to low oxygen or high carbon dioxide levels. But a study done in 1987 subjected volunteers to high oxygen levels and found that they certainly did not yawn less, and nor did high carbon dioxide levels make them yawn more. Other theories suggest that yawning stretches out the lungs and nearby tissues, preventing tiny airways in the lungs from collapsing and developing chest infections, or that it helps to distribute a chemical called surfactant, which coats the lungs, helping to keep them open.

As to why yawning is contagious, it's probably the power of suggestion that leads one person to yawn after seeing someone else do so. This may be an involuntary, genetically programmed phenomenon: once one person in the 'tribe' yawned, others did so because this behaviour pattern helped our evolutionary ancestors to communicate with one another.

Why do we have eyebrows?

Anthropologists think eyebrows are important for forming facial expressions that can be easily recognized even at a distance by other individuals in one's social group. They also serve the practical purpose of stopping sweat and rain running down your forehead into your eyes.

What does your appendix do?

There are a few theories. One is that it is a vestigial structure, a reminder of a large, more fully functioning organ that humans used to have, but that has now long since evolved away. Another theory, proposed by Charles Darwin, is that the appendix was previously used for digesting leaves and cellulose from tree bark, etc. Today humans can't digest this roughage, but Darwin thought perhaps we once could.

A more likely theory is that it aids recovery from diarrhoea. An infection enters the guts and the resulting diarrhoea and overload of pathogenic bugs wipes out the 'good bacteria' in the intestines. The theory suggests that only the appendix remains untouched by the infection and so contains a reserve of good bacteria which can recolonize the gut once the infection has subsided.

Did You Know... The human body is estimated to have 60,000 miles of blood vessels. To put that in perspective, the distance around the Earth is about 25,000 miles, making the distance your blood vessels could travel if laid end to end more than two times around the Earth.

Why does food taste so bland when you have a cold and blocked nose? Do we need smell to taste?

With your nose blocked up you can still taste sweet, salty, savoury, sour and bitter. Taste buds on your tongue detect the flavours dissolved in saliva while eating. But that's all. You won't be able to detect any subtle flavours, which is why food tastes bland when you are bunged up. To detect these you do need air flowing through your nasal pathways, to carry taste chemicals to the olfactory receptors just under the brain, behind the bridge of your nose. We only taste five different 'flavours', but we can detect around 10,000 different smells. That's still a lot less than many other animals, like the rat, who can distinguish between 30,000 and 100,000 different smells.

What are blood groups and why do we have them?

Blood is made up of four main components: red blood cells, white blood cells, platelets, and plasma. There are different types of blood because each red blood cell has special chemical markers called antigens on it. Antigens are types of proteins, glycoproteins and glycolipids on the surface of red blood cells, and are what define blood types. Sophisticated biochemistry and molecular biology research techniques have helped us to characterize a number of the surface proteins. Although it appears that the majority of them are not actually essential for red cell function, some have specific functions such as allowing substances to enter and exit the red cell or binding certain substances to the cell surface.

Your blood type is inherited from your biological parents, in a similar way to eye or hair colour. Karl Landsteiner described the original blood types A, B and O in 1900, but doctors now recognize 23 blood group systems with hundreds of different 'types'.

We know that for some blood types, evolution and environmental selective pressures are clearly important for their persistence. For example, the percentage of people lacking a particular antigen called the Duffy antigen is much higher in certain parts of Africa. The reason is to do with malaria. The Duffy blood type includes a receptor that allows certain types of malarial parasites to enter the red cell. So in some malarial areas of Africa, populations with Duffy-negative blood types have a distinct survival advantage, because absence of the Duffy antigen provides a measure of protection against malaria.

We don't yet know the functions of the A and B blood groups (blood group O indicates simply the absence of A and B factors), but there are differences in the rate at which certain cancers occur within the different groups: people with blood group A have about a 20 per cent greater risk of developing cancer of the stomach than people with blood group O, who in turn appear to have a greater risk of developing ulcers. The reasons again are unclear. There is some evidence that group Os are more susceptible than other blood types to the agent that causes bubonic plague, whereas group A people are more susceptible to smallpox virus. These correlations may account for the increased frequency of the B group in China, India and parts of Russia, which suffered epidemics of both of these diseases.

Did You Know… The surface area of a human lung is equal to a tennis court.

What happens when we fall in love?

The science of love is very complex and not well understood, but is certainly due to chemicals released in our brain when we are drawn to someone. One of these, phenylethylamine, makes us feel very excited and that everything is wonderful. In the next stage of love, a hormone called oxytocin is released. This plays an important role throughout our lives: it is a 'cuddle hormone' and acts as a kind of infatuation chemical. Childbirth and the noise of a baby crying also make it flow, which helps parents to bond and feel protective towards their children. Beyond these it is still very much one of life's wonderful mysteries.

Does cracking your knuckles really give you arthritis?

Another popular myth, this one probably started to dissuade people from doing it as it is so annoying. It may make your joints sore but there's no evidence that it causes arthritis. If you crack your knuckles all the time, however, you could injure the cartilage and cause the joints to swell. Keep this up and eventually it might lead to degenerative joint disease, such as arthritis, but the occasional crack will do no harm, only irritate those next to you.

Top 10 Preserved Body Parts of Historical Figures

1) Einstein's Brain
Removed during his autopsy and without his family's permission, Einstein's brain was dissected and examined for a cause of his genius. Parts of the brain were sent to scientists all around the world.

2) Hitler's Penis
When Russian soldiers discovered and mutilated Hitler's body, one soldier, Vasily Zudropov, kept the Fuhrer's member, preserved it and passed it on to his son. It remains in the Zudropov family collection. Other preserved penises of the famous include Napoleon's and Rasputin's, although in the latter case some experts think that rather than being the phallus of the mad monk it is actually the preserved specimen of a sea cucumber. It is impressively large.

3) Galileo's Finger
Known as the father of modern science, after his death Galileo's finger was removed and is displayed in the Galileo Museum in Florence, Italy. Perhaps in a final ironic gesture to the Catholic Church it is his middle finger that stands upright in defiance. Galileo was right, the world does revolve round the sun, but the church imprisoned him for stating this.

4) George Washington's Hair
Despite having wooden teeth, it was actually President Washington's hair that was kept after his death. Requested by the aunt of the poet Henry Wadsworth Longfellow, it was later donated to the Maine Historical Society.

5) Jeremy Bentham's Head
Philosopher and founder of University College London, Bentham actually requested that his body be dissected as part of a public anatomy lecture. Afterwards, the skeleton and head were preserved and stored in a wooden cabinet, with the skeleton stuffed out with hay and dressed in Bentham's clothes. Called an 'auto-icon', it is now on display in University College and used during board meetings. It has become the target of repeated student pranks, including being stolen on more than one occasion.

6) Spallanzani's Bladder
An Italian biologist who proved that sexual reproduction involves a sperm and an egg and who also performed the world's first-ever successful artificial insemination, his bladder is preserved and on display in the University History Museum in Pavia, Italy.

7) The Buddha's Tooth
Apparently taken from the Buddha's funeral pyre in India, this religious artefact has a whole temple dedicated to it in Sri Lanka.

There are vast numbers of supposed body parts of saints in existence, including what are claimed to be several preserved samples of the foreskin of Christ and no fewer than two skulls belonging to John the Baptist – the explanation for these being that one is from John as a young man, the other was taken after he was decapitated.

8) Dan Sickles' Leg
A Union general who lost his leg to a cannonball at the Battle of Gettysburg during the US Civil War, Sickles fought on bravely until the leg had to be amputated later that day. Sickles' leg, and a replica of the cannonball that shattered it, are displayed at the American National Museum of Health and Medicine in Washington, DC.

9) Paul Broca's Brain
French physician and anthropologist Paul Broca is best known for his mid-1800s discovery of the speech production centre of the brain in the frontal lobe, now known as Broca's area. His brain is on display at the Museum of Man in Paris.

10) Saint Catherine Laboure's Body
Saint Catherine Laboure died on 31st December 1876. When her body was exhumed 56 years later it was unblemished and undecomposed. Her eyes were as blue as the day she died. Catherine Laboure is still lying in state at the right of the altar in the chapel Rue du Bac 140 in Paris, and she still looks as though she died only yesterday.

Do copper bracelets really help arthritis sufferers?

They are sold everywhere, and all come with claims that they can relieve the pain and swelling of rheumatoid arthritis. Unfortunately, such claims are more designed to sell the product than to provide you with sound medical advice. To be fair to users, the bracelets have been around for centuries, even used by the ancient Greeks. There is actually some truth to the idea that copper may play a small role in pain relief: some animal studies have shown that taking copper by mouth may reduce the progression of joint and tissue damage in arthritis sufferers, and gold forms part of several prescription medications for arthritis. Unfortunately, the use of copper bracelets for arthritis hasn't been shown to have the same effect in scientific studies.

There is some evidence that copper has both antioxidant and pro-oxidant effects depending on copper levels in the body. (Antioxidants such as the vitamins A, C and E fight the damage caused by oxidization in the body.) If it does exhibit antioxidant properties, there's the possibility it could have a limited, positive effect on arthritis symptoms, although there are many foods that have a higher antioxidant potential without the negative pro-oxidant effect. But so far researchers have found that copper and magnetic bracelets are useless. No differences in perceived pain were found when copper strips, magnetic strips or placebo strips were tested against each other. It appears that any perceived benefit obtained from wearing a magnetic or copper bracelet can be attributed to psychological placebo effects. Funny, then, that this should have become a multimillion-pound alternative pain therapy industry.

Did You Know... Scientists have counted over 500 different liver functions. It's one of the body's hardest-working and biggest organs. Just some of the functions your liver performs include production of bile, decomposition of red blood cells, plasma protein synthesis, and detoxification.

If you sneeze with your eyes open will they fall out?

No! Your eyes are held in your head by six strong muscles, and will not go flying out if you sneeze with them open. People came up with this nonsense probably because it seems impossible not to close your eyes when you sneeze. And if we can't force our own eyes to stay open during a sneeze, then, so the theory went, there must therefore be a good reason for them to shut involuntarily. Not necessarily. It's probably just an involuntary reaction with no real purpose. The eyes may close during a sneeze for the same reason your leg kicks out when your knee is tapped.

And it's not just the muscles in your eyelids that react during a sneeze. Many muscles all over your body react. For example, many people with stress incontinence experience urine leakages when they sneeze – the result of those muscles tensing and releasing involuntarily.

Does reading in dim light really damage your eyes?

Children are frequently issued the ominous warning that reading by torchlight under the bed covers will ruin their eyes. It's not true, however. Reading in low light does not damage eyes, but rather causes eyestrain instead.

When you walk into a room where light is low, your eye adjusts in several ways. First, the rod and cone cells on the retina begin to produce more light-sensitive chemicals. These chemicals detect light, convert it to an electrical signal and transmit that signal to the brain. Second, the iris muscles relax, which causes the opening of your eye, the pupil, to become very large. This allows your eye to collect as much light as possible. Finally, the nerve cells in the retina adapt so that they can work in low light. If you read in low light, your visual muscles get mixed signals: relax to collect the most light, but at the same time contract to maintain the focused image. When that object is poorly lit, focusing becomes even more difficult because the contrast between the words and the page isn't as great, which decreases the eye's ability to distinguish visual detail. That ability is called *visual acuity*. Your eyes have to work harder to separate the words from the page, which strains your eye muscles.

When your eyes are working this hard for a long period of time, they become tired, much as any muscle would. The strain may result in a number of physical effects including sore or itching eyeballs, headaches, back and neck aches and blurred vision.

But this won't damage your eyes, and will go away when you stop reading and rest them.

What are goosebumps?

Tiny muscles in our skin contract, causing the hairs to stand on end. They also cause a slight tethering of the skin, creating raised bumps around the hair follicles: goosebumps. This helps to trap air in a layer all over our bodies and so keep us warm. Obviously since we have become less hairy creatures this is not as effective as it was when we proudly sported a thick covering of body hair. The raised hairs also make us look bigger (think about cats raising their fur when threatened) and therefore stronger – a defence mechanism that may explain why we get goosebumps when scared.

Is it true that our stomach acid is as strong as battery acid?

The acid in your stomach is strong enough to dissolve razorblades. While you certainly shouldn't test the fortitude of your stomach by eating a razorblade (or any other metal object, for that matter), the acids that digest the food you eat aren't to be taken lightly. Hydrochloric acid, the type found in your stomach, is not only good at dissolving the pizza you had for dinner but can also eat through many types of metal.

You get a new stomach lining every three to four days. The mucus-like cells lining the walls of the stomach would soon dissolve due to the strong digestive acids in your stomach if they weren't constantly replaced. Those with ulcers know how painful it can be when stomach acid takes its toll on the deeper layers of the lining of your stomach.

Did You Know... The aorta is nearly the diameter of a garden hose. The average adult heart is about the size of two fists, making the size of the aorta quite impressive. The artery needs to be so large as it is the main supplier of rich, oxygenated blood to the rest of the body.

How many organs could we have removed and still survive?

You could actually survive with surprisingly few organs left intact. You could remove the stomach, the spleen, 75 per cent of the liver, 80 per cent of the intestines, one kidney, one lung and virtually every organ from the pelvic and groin area and still live. You might not feel too great, but not having those organs wouldn't kill you.

Sometimes when I'm staring at a wall or the sky I can see specks and little thread-like things floating by. They move when I move my eyes, and I have friends who say that they get them, too. What on earth are they and should I be worried?

Those little specks and threads that you can see are inside your eyeball, within the jelly-like substance that fills the inside. We doctors call them floaters, and the really brainy ones among us call them *muscae volitantes*.

Pretty much everyone experiences them, although they're most common in people who are short sighted. It's thought that the little threads are remnants of the hyaloid artery, which supplies the lens and other parts of the eye during foetal development but then is no longer required and so withers away. It runs from the lens to the back of the eye during early development, and starts to atrophy after the third month. Most of the debris has disappeared by the time you are born, but some of it remains indefinitely.

The number of floaters in your eyes tends to increase with age, due to the formation of fibrous clumps and membranes in the vitreous fluid. I should add that floaters aren't always totally benign. Sometimes they can result from blood cells released into the eyeball from a haemorrhage of the delicate vessels inside the eye, possibly following a trauma, and a sudden increase of spots, often with flashes of light, can herald a detached retina. In your case they sound quite harmless and normal, however.

Did You Know... Your left lung is smaller than your right lung to make room for your heart, which is tilted slightly to the left, making it take up more room on that side of the body and crowding out the left lung.

Do we really only use 10 per cent of our brains?

Even though we are still in the dark about many of the exact functional details of parts of the brain, we do know that every part of the brain has a known function. This oft-quoted myth about only using 10 per cent of our brains probably arose from a misunderstanding or misinterpretation of some neurological research done in the late 1800s and early 1900s, which reported that only about 10 per cent of the neurons in the brain are firing at any given time. The same researchers also explained how they had only managed to map the functions of 10 per cent of the brain. But this certainly doesn't mean that the other areas are not used.

There is a reason for the sparing use of neurons: if all of a person's neurons began firing at once, that person would not become a genius, but would instead suffer a major seizure.

Further confusion may arise from the fact that only 10 per cent of the cells in the brain are neurons. The rest are called glial cells, and do not function in the same way as neurons.

To put the myth to bed completely, MRI imaging has clearly shown that humans put most of their cerebral cortex to good use, even while sleeping.

You can't grow new brain cells, right? You continually lose them throughout your life.

This is not true. New neurons can grow within a mature adult brain, a process known as *neurogenesis*. A new study has shown that neurons continue to grow and change beyond the first years of development and well into adulthood.

New neurons are born in predominantly two regions of the brain: the subventricular zone lining the lateral ventricles, where the new cells migrate to the smell receptors, and in the subgranular zone of the hippocampus.

Many of these newborn cells die shortly after their birth, but a number of them become functionally integrated into the surrounding brain tissue.

Did You Know... Your brain uses 20 per cent of the oxygen that enters your bloodstream. The brain only makes up about 2 per cent of our body mass, yet consumes more oxygen than any other organ in the body, making it extremely susceptible to damage related to oxygen deprivation.

Is there any connection between the size of a man's feet and the size of his penis?

My old university, UCL, has looked into this popular rumour. They measured the feet and penises of over 100 men and found that the average penis was 13 cm (5 inches) when soft, within a range of 6 cm (2.5 inches) at the lower end of the scale to 18 cm (7.5 inches) at the higher end. The average British male shoe size is 9 (or 43 in European measurements). The study found *no* correlation at all between shoe size and penis length.

Did You Know... Your brain cannot feel pain. While the brain might be the pain centre when you cut your finger or burn yourself, the brain itself does not have pain receptors and so cannot feel pain if injured.

Skin, Hair & Nails

I have lots of moles all over my body. Does this mean I am more at risk of cancer? What are the warning signs?

Moles are simply an overgrowth of the pigment cells within the deeper layer of the skin. Virtually everyone has some. Statistically, you'll find between 10 and 50 moles on the average body, and they can occur on any part of the body.

Interestingly, it is thought that we are born with all the moles we will ever have. Many of them are not visible at birth but will darken with age and with sun exposure, and appear on those areas that get most sunlight.

The main problem is that a small number of these moles can develop into a form of skin cancer called *malignant melanoma*. Having large numbers of moles (more than 25) may mean you are more susceptible to melanoma, so you should take great care about exposure to sunlight. If people in your family have had melanoma, then you should check your moles carefully. Avoid too much sun, particularly the two hours either side of midday, and avoid getting sunburn. If you got burnt a lot when you were younger then your risk of skin cancer will be much higher. Warning signs are any changes to the moles, so be vigilant and ask your GP if you are not sure.

My life is plagued by my sweat problem – I'm always wet with sweat. Is there anything I can do about it?

Excessive sweating can be a really embarrassing problem. You don't just have to be too hot – nerves and stressful situations can get you soaked through in no time. In women there can be a hormonal element to it, too. You may need to try a prescription-strength anti-perspirant containing aluminium salts, or there are some medications available that block the effect of the nerves that stimulate the glands. These pills don't work for everyone, however, and can have side-effects. An operation to cut the nerve supply to the sweat glands is also available, but again may not work every time. It can cause a reactive increase in sweating in another part of the body in some people.

A more modern treatment involves Botox injections to paralyse the sweat glands, but you may need a lot of these before it works well and it only lasts for 4 to 12 months.

Some general advice: avoid any triggers such as heat or spicy foods, and choose black or white clothes that won't show the sweat so much.

Did You Know... Feet have 500,000 sweat glands and can produce more than a pint of sweat a day.

I've had psoriasis for some time, and I have now developed painful lumps on my hands and feet that hurt when I walk. I smoke but am otherwise healthy. Is there anything I can do to help it?

You may have something called palmo-plantar pustulosis, which is a nasty type of psoriasis that causes pustules on the palms of the hands and soles of the feet. The first things you should do is stop smoking, as you may have an abnormal response to nicotine which can trigger flares of your psoriasis.

There are many different treatments around including some new breakthrough drugs that seem to be effective. An acne medication called isotretinoin (Roaccutane) and a couple of new drugs called tacrolimus and pimecrolimus seem to work well. Ask your GP for a referral to a dermatologist, who can explain the options to you.

Does eating chocolate give you spots?

Loads of studies have been done on the connection between diet and acne, and none has found any link at all. Acne is caused by hormones, and is made worse by stress, and that is all there is to it. Greasy food, junk food, sweets and chocolate are not responsible. Your mother just told you that to stop you eating so much.

Is it true that shaving causes hair to grow back faster, thicker and darker?

This is a rumour that is convenient for the hair-removal industry, but it's not true. Shaving will not make hair grow back thicker, or any faster. It's an illusion created because the hair grows back blunt-ended without the fine tapered ends of unshaven hair, and so looks and feels thicker. Furthermore, the sun naturally bleaches hair over time, so hair that is newly emerged may seem darker but is, in fact, no darker than any other new hair growth.

Did You Know... It takes 17 muscles to smile and 43 to frown. Unless you're trying to give your face a bit of a workout, smiling is a much easier option for most of us.

My friends say I have acne because I am dirty and don't wash properly. Is this really true?

Many people think acne is caused by dirty skin and even a poor diet, but this is simply not true. Acne is the direct manifestation of the production of hormones, which explains why it is so prevalent in teenagers. Treatment involves prescription drugs. That is not to suggest, however, that in some people a vast improvement in diet wouldn't have a noticeable impact on their skin.

I wear my hair in a tight ponytail but my mum says it could make me bald – how can this be?

Hairstyles such as tight ponytails, plaits or corn-rows can cause hair loss due to the constant tension they subject the hair to, which gradually pulls hairs out. Winding hair tightly onto heated rollers can have the same damaging effect. Hair extensions, if put in too tightly, can cause bald patches, as many celebrities are now finding out.

Does stress make your hair go grey quicker?

Stress is blamed for a huge variety of illnesses, and in many cases it is partly responsible, especially in the case of heart disease, headaches, stomach problems, sleep disorders and a compromised immune system, to name just a few. Stress can also cause exacerbations of acne or psoriasis, and trigger conditions like telogen effluvium or alopecia areata, both of which cause hair to fall out.

But can stress turn hair grey? This theory probably arose from reports that Marie Antoinette showed up for her execution with grey hair; it was believed that her hair colour changed overnight as she waited, in fear, for her fate. But this was more likely to have been due to the fact that she no longer had on an elaborate wig, nor had had access to hair dye for some time before her execution.

Going grey is a normal part of ageing: about 50 per cent of 50-year-olds are halfway to grey. Grey hairs usually start appearing between the ages of 30 and 35, but the rate of greying differs according to factors such as race.

Stress can cause hair loss, and so it's possible that losing some pigmented hair can make any grey hairs more noticeable, but it doesn't make the hair go grey. No direct link between stress and grey hair has been found.

If you want to figure out when you'll go grey, you need look no further than your parents – it's our genes that have the power over what comes out of each hair follicle.

The results of a 2009 Japanese study did indicate that genotoxic stress, in the form of ultraviolet light and chemicals, damages our DNA and could cause the depletion of pigment in our hair. There is not much you can do about this, however, as researchers estimate that just one mammalian cell is subjected to 100,000 such stressors in any given day.

One last theory about grey hair is that it occurs due to the amount of hydrogen peroxide in our follicles that builds up over time. It's early days in this research, however, so for now I would suggest that when it comes to grey hair, there may be no way to escape your genetic destiny.

Did You Know... I'm not sure if blondes really do have more fun, but they certainly have more hair. Hair colour determines how dense the hair on your head is. The average human has 100,000 hair follicles; blondes average 146,000 follicles, while people with black hair tend to have about 110,000 follicles. Those with brown hair fit the average, with 100,000 follicles, and redheads have the least dense hair, with about 86,000 follicles.

Is it true that too much blow-drying and heated brushes can worsen hair loss?

True. The reason is that extreme heat damages the proteins in the hairs, making them fragile and liable to break off. Brushing the hair during blow-drying causes even more damage. Careless use of heated brushes or heated hair straighteners can even burn the scalp, so that the hair follicles are permanently damaged in that area.

I always buy expensive protein-containing conditioners and shampoos that promise to nourish my hair and help it to grow, but my sister laughs at me and says they are a waste of money. Is she right?

Well, look at it this way: protein-containing conditioners only temporarily fill in defects on the surface of the hair shaft, making it smoother and thicker so your hair will *look* good, but the shampoos will not help it grow or 'nourish' it. Hair is a dead tissue.

Top 10 Best Foods

1) Sweet Potatoes
A nutritional concentrate and quite possibly one of the best vegetables you can eat. Loaded with carotenoids, vitamin C, potassium and fibre, use them instead of normal potatoes for a healthier choice.

2) Grape Tomatoes
Sweeter and firmer than other tomatoes, and perfect for snacking, dipping or salads, they are packed with vitamins C and A.

3) Fat-free or Very Low-fat Milk
While I personally prefer soymilk, cow's milk is an excellent source of calcium, vitamins and protein with little or no artery-clogging fat and cholesterol. The same applies to low-fat yogurt. Soymilk can be just as nutritious if it is fortified.

4) Broccoli
Packed with vitamin C, carotenoids and folic acid. Steam it just til it's still firm and add a squeeze of lemon juice.

5) Wild Salmon
The omega-3 fats in fatty fish like salmon can help reduce the risk of sudden-death heart attacks.

6) Crispbreads
Possibly an odd choice for my list, you may think, but wholegrain rye crackers are loaded with fibre and are fat-free.

7) Microwave Quick-cook Brown Rice
These microwaveable packs of brown rice are easy to prepare and more nutritious than enriched white rice. Brown rice contains

more fibre, magnesium, vitamins E and B$_6$, copper, zinc and phytochemicals than white rice.

8) Citrus Fruits

Rich in vitamin C, folic acid and fibre, and available in many different types: juicy Minneola oranges, clementines, tangerines, blood oranges and tart pink grapefruit – although be careful with eating grapefruit if you are on certain medications.

9) Diced Butternut Squash

Steam a sliced squash or buy sliced butternut squash that's ready to go into the oven or into a stir-fry or soup. They are an easy way to get loads of vitamins A and C and fibre.

10) Spinach and Kale

These leafy greens are jam-packed with vitamins A, C and K, folate, potassium, magnesium, iron, lutein and phytochemicals. Serve with a spritz of lemon juice.

My father has a full head of hair, so does this mean that I will not go bald?

No. A tendency to baldness is inherited from both parents and probably involves a combination of genes. So you are not automatically in the clear even if your father has a full head of hair. It is not true, as is sometimes claimed, that only genes from the mother's side are involved.

My doctor told me that being bald means that you are more likely to have a heart attack, and now I'm worried. Is he right?

He is, to some extent. A study has found that men who had lost hair at the crown of their heads had a 40 per cent increased chance of heart disease. Hair loss at the front of the head (a receding hairline) increased the risk by 28 per cent. So if you have 'male pattern baldness' you should stop smoking, eat healthily, have your blood pressure checked and do some exercise.

Did You Know... About 32 million bacteria call every inch of your skin home. The majority of these are entirely harmless and some are even helpful in maintaining a healthy body.

At 15 I got bad acne on my face. It has now spread across my chest and back in hard, red, painful lumps that look awful. I've tried all the stuff you can get in chemists' shops but they haven't helped. Will I ever get rid of it?

Acne is one of the more distressing conditions to have, and strikes in the teen years when you are at your most sensitive and most concerned about the way you look. It needs to be taken seriously as it can leave you with permanent scars. It has nothing whatsoever to do with cleanliness, or with what you eat. Chocolate and fatty foods don't make it worse, although there is some evidence that milk may do in some people.

The good news is that acne can be successfully treated. There is a very effective treatment that you are certainly a good candidate for. It's called Roaccutane. You have to take it every day as a pill. It has some serious side-effects, including drying of the skin and eyes and can give you really cracked, sore lips. It can also affect your liver and you should have blood tests while on the treatment. It really does work, though, and I would ask your GP about it. You may need to be on it for about six months, and you won't really notice any changes until you have been on it for two to three months or so. It reduces scarring and stops those painful red boils that you are getting now.

Why does hair turn grey? Do dark-haired people turn grey earlier, or is it only more noticeable?

The process of going grey is not very well understood. One thing we know for sure is that there is no correlation between greyness and balding, another common myth.

Your hair colour is determined by the pigment melanin that is distributed through the middle of the hair shaft. The actual final colour depends on the number, size and colour of the pigment granules. The lighter someone's hair, the less melanin there is. Brown or black hair has much more melanin than blond or red. Skin colour often goes with hair colour, too. For some reason the cells that manufacture melanin can slow down or stop completely. This causes the hair to lose its colour, turning yellow and then grey. Air bubbles, which may mysteriously work their way into the hair shaft, also contribute to greying by blocking the passage of the melanin. It seems to be genetically determined, and the process is the same for light- and dark-haired people, but the pigment loss is indeed more obvious in darker hairs.

Did You Know... Human hair is virtually indestructible. Aside from its flammability, human hair decays at such a slow rate that it is practically non-disintegrative. Hair cannot be destroyed by cold, change of climate, water or other natural forces, and it is resistant to many kinds of acids and corrosive chemicals.

My nails have ridges in them. They look horrible, even with nail polish on them. Why do they grow like this, and what can I do?

Ridges in nails are not unusual and can be a sign of general illness. A single lengthwise ridge could be due to a cyst or growth in the nail bed, while crosswise ridges may be due to eczema, recurrent nail bed infections, keeping your nails wet all the time (for example if you do lots of washing up or hand laundry), and the habit of pulling back the quick at the base of the nails. You can get lengthwise ridges in your nails if you have poor circulation to your fingers; these are common in the elderly. A single crosswise ridge is called a Beau's line, and you can get this after being really unwell or stressed for a time.

Treatment depends on the type of ridges you have, so I suggest you show your doctor so he or she can help you work out which problem yours is.

My feet have got really itchy, especially between my toes. They smell more, too, and the skin looks whitish and wrinkled like I have just got out of a long bath. What could be wrong?

I bet you wear trainers a lot. You probably have something called athlete's foot. It's caused by a fungal infection of the skin and makes it really itchy and boggy-looking, just like you describe. You can catch it from other people in gyms and swimming pools, but it is not serious and is quite easy to treat, too. Just go to a chemist and buy some over-the-counter cream like Lamisil. You can also get sprays and powders, so go for whatever appeals to you most. It may be wise to invest in a new pair of trainers and try to go around barefoot as much as you can at home; this will help your feet dry out and stop you getting more infections.

Did You Know... Like fingerprints, every tongue print is also unique.

I've got really bad dandruff and can't wear black clothes at all any more. Is there anything I can do to control it?

Dandruff, caused by excessive shedding of dead skin, doesn't usually require any medical treatment, but yours sounds severe. If you also get some redness and inflammation on your scalp then you may have a condition called seborrheic dermatitis and should see your GP. To treat it you need to shampoo regularly with over-the-counter dandruff shampoos containing ingredients such as coal tar, salicylic acid and zinc pyrithione (an antifungal agent).

My mother always told me that having white spots in your nails was a sign of not enough calcium in the diet. Is there any truth in this?

Actually there is not, although a lot of people do believe this. My mother used to tell me the same thing! Irregular white spots in your nails are, more often than not, caused by minor trauma sustained while that part of the nail was forming. This usually involves some sort of impact damage to the nail bed. They may take some time to appear, as nails grow slowly, so the actual event itself is usually long forgotten.

Totally white nails are something different and can indicate malnutrition or liver disease, so probably best to get this checked out by your GP – but they're nothing to do with calcium, however.

Do your nails all grow at the same speed? I'm sure I need to cut some of mine more often than others.

They don't all grow at the same speed. Fingernails grow nearly four times faster than toenails. If you notice that you're trimming your fingernails much more frequently than your toenails, you're not just imagining it. And it doesn't end there. The fastest growing nail is on the middle finger. And the nail on the middle finger of your dominant hand will grow the fastest of all. Why is not entirely known. It may be because the nail on the middle finger of your dominant hand is the one most likely to wear down fastest. We do know that nail growth is related to the length of the fingers: the longest fingers grow nails the fastest, the shortest the slowest.

Did You Know... There are at least five types of receptors in the skin that respond to pain and to touch.

I have extremely sensitive skin: if I scratch or bump myself, even lightly, my skin comes up in raised red welts. Why is this?

What you are describing sounds like a classic case of *dermographia*. This is a condition characterized by an excessive reaction to pressure on the skin, resulting in a localized attack of hives (urticaria) at the point where you are scratched or bumped. It can be extremely annoying if it is very severe. It can develop at any age and is far more common in women than men. You have probably found that the red welts come up in a few minutes, but can take several hours or even days to fade away.

There is no permanent cure, but you could try taking antihistamine tablets on a regular basis to reduce the severity of the reaction.

Some sufferers have used their condition to turn their bodies into living works of art, lightly scraping patterns and designs over their skin, which then form the red lesions, and some have written pages of religious texts over their bodies.

My daughter has just been started on treatment for ringworm. How did she catch these worms?

Ringworm is not a worm at all, but a fungal infection of the skin. It's caught from another body, be it human or animal, which already has the disease. The fungal spore that causes the disease penetrates into the skin, and starts growing there. It causes a small red spot that gradually gets bigger and then develops a pale centre. As the fungus grows, the edge of the spreading infection becomes red and inflamed, while the area that has recovered returns to a normal skin colour. Thus a slowly enlarging ring appears. This is a very typical growth pattern for fungi: you see the same phenomenon when toadstools grow in wet grass, forming a ring.

Why do I have loads of rough little bumps all over the backs of my arms? Quite a few of my school friends have them, too. How can we get rid of them?

This is a very common genetic condition of the hair follicles called *keratosis pilaris*, or *follicular keratosis*. It most often appears on the back and outer sides of the upper arms, and can also occur on the thighs, hands, tops of the legs, flanks, buttocks – any body part except the palms or the soles of the feet.

The condition is surprisingly common, which is why some of your friends have it, and it's estimated that it affects around 40 per cent of the adult population and 50–80 per cent of all adolescents. It is also more common in men than in women, and is often worse in cold, dry weather.

It occurs because of excess keratin production, which surrounds and entraps the hair follicles in the affected area. This causes hard plugs to form, which make up those bumps that you can feel. The bumps can also contain a coiled up in-growing hair.

Unfortunately there is no cure for keratosis pilaris, but there are treatments available including vitamin A-derivative creams, adapalene, benzoyl peroxide and triamcinolone. These can all help the appearance and texture of the skin, but you should know that once therapy is discontinued, the condition reverts to its original state.

Exfoliation, intensive moisturizers, alpha-hydroxy acids and urea may be of help, too.

Did You Know... Three hundred million cells die in the human body every minute, but this is just a small fraction of the total cells that are in your body. Estimates have placed the total number of cells in the body at 10–50 trillion.

Bowels & Bottoms

Does being stressed give you ulcers?

Doctors used to think that a peptic ulcer was the result of too much stress or spicy food, or both. However, Nobel Prize-winning research pinned the blame on a bacteria called *Helicobacter pylori*, a spiral-shaped organism that causes more than 90 per cent of ulcers and thrives in highly acid conditions. It does its damage by weakening the protective mucus coating of the stomach and duodenum that normally protects us from corrosive stomach acid. If weakened by the bacteria, this mucus shield is rendered ineffective, allowing acid to get through to the sensitive lining underneath. While it's not clear how people pick up the *H. pylori* infection in the first place, researchers suspect that it's from person-to-person contact, either through infected saliva, vomit or faecal matter that comes into contact with hands, food or water.

The stress link is not totally irrelevant, though: stress can increase gastric acidity and acid production, and so make the damage worse.

Not every ulcer is caused this way, however. Certain drugs like non-steroidal anti-inflammatory drugs (NSAIDs), such as ibuprofen or aspirin, can have a similar effect, weakening the mucus coating and so making the person taking them prone to developing ulcers. In much rarer cases, cancerous tumours in the stomach or pancreas can cause ulcers.

I have a really itchy bottom and it is driving me crazy. I have tried pile cream from various GPs and that doesn't seem to work. Is there anything else I can do?

This is a much more common problem than you might think, especially with people who sit a lot, such as lorry and cab drivers. The reason that it seems to go on and on is due to something called the 'scratch–itch cycle'. This is essentially where you scratch around your bum because it is itching, but this scratching breaks the skin slightly. Superficial inflammation and infection can then occur, which only makes the itch worse. You scratch it again and the cycle continues. To break this cycle it is important to treat any skin infection that may be present, using antibiotic tablets or skin-cleaning creams.

Avoid adding things to the bathwater such as bubble bath, and always pat yourself dry there rather than rubbing vigorously with a towel.

Keep in mind things like threadworms, which are a common cause of itchy bottoms, especially at night. If you live with young children you may have picked threadworms up from them. They are easily treated with an over-the-counter medication.

Did You Know... The large intestine is 7 to 10 cm wide. The large intestine is divided into six pieces, called the caecum, ascending colon, transverse colon, descending colon, sigmoid colon, and the rectum. Food in the large intestine can remain there for between 18 hours and 2 days.

My husband is suffering from anal fissures and is in terrible pain. We would like to know how to treat this problem.

Fissures are small tears in the tissue at the opening of the anus. They can be very sore and sting when having a bowel movement. Treatments consist of trying to prevent constipation, because straining to pass the stool and passing large, hard stools cause more problems. Laxatives can be used for a short time to give the fissure a chance to heal. The only other medical treatments are certain types of suppositories or creams to be applied locally, which help to relax the muscles of the bottom and aid healing. In more resistant cases, surgery might be recommended.

Should I be concerned that I only go for a poo about once a week? I have always been like this.

There is no 'normal' bowel habit. Most people go between three times a day and twice a week on average. If you have always gone to the loo with this frequency then it's clearly normal for you, but any changes to your bowel habit should always been investigated by a doctor. One of the symptoms of bowel cancer is an altered bowel habit, with alternating periods of constipation and diarrhoea.

I was diagnosed with glandular fever about three weeks ago. I feel fine now and want to get back to playing rugby, but I keep hearing that this could be dangerous if your spleen is enlarged. Do I need to worry about this and get a scan or something?

This is a very sensible question to ask. Your spleen is found under the left-hand side of your abdomen, tucked up out of the way under your ribs for protection. During an attack of glandular fever your spleen can become enlarged and can protrude down below the edge of the rib cage, making it more exposed and vulnerable to impacts to that area.

You shouldn't need to have any sort of scan to find out if your spleen has got bigger, however. Your doctor can examine you to find this out without too much difficulty. If your spleen cannot be felt, then it was either never enlarged or it has been enlarged but has now gone back to a more normal size. If your doctor can feel your spleen, then you should not play rugby until it has settled down again.

Top 10 Most Crippling Phobias

1) Domatophobia

For most of us the basic idea of security is having four walls, three meals a day and a bed to sleep on. For sufferers of domatophobia, these basic life necessities form the basis of their crippling phobia: fear of houses or being in a house.

2) Urophobia

You can probably guess this means a fear of urination. It can arise from no obvious source or be learned from a traumatic experience like a painful bladder infection or herpes outbreak. Sometimes a catheter has to be used to avoid the anxiety around actually going to the toilet.

3) Decidophobia

I'm not making these up, I promise. Decidophobia is the fear of making decisions. A person who cannot make a decision is likely to be eternally stuck in a rut. Unless something becomes second nature, such as everyday routines, a sufferer may well be crippled by the simple decision of what to eat for breakfast. And before you ask, no, it's not found commonly in women!

4) Nyctophobia and Photophobia

Two similar but opposite phobias. One is the fear of night or darkness, the other the fear of light.

5) Somniphobia and Clinophobia

You don't necessarily have to be clinophobic to be somniphobic. A person with somniphobia fears sleep, while a person suffering from clinophobia fears beds. Humans need the REM cycles of sleep to help process their everyday thoughts and activities, and without sleep a person could suffer serious mental breakdown. This is why these two phobias are particularly crippling.

6) Chronophobia

The fear of clocks or even the fear of time itself. The thought that time is constantly slipping away can cause sanity to do so as well.

7) Stasibasiphobia

A fear of standing up and walking. A person with stasibasiphobia finds it virtually impossible to carry out any life functions unless confined to a wheelchair. Some are even phobic of others standing and walking, too, an obviously crippling phobia.

8) Anthropophobia and Lalophobia

These two fears could potentially isolate the phobic for life. Anthropophobia is a fear of people, while lalophobia is the fear of speaking. Makes holding down a job, having a family or any sort of social life virtually impossible.

9) Phagophobia

Something most definitely not seen widely enough in the US: phagophobia is the fear of eating. Occasionally seen in children and sometimes a sign of an autistic spectrum disorder, it may be grouped with disorders like anorexia nervosa.

10) Anemophobia

Incredibly, this means a fear of air, and can leaving sufferers scared every moment of their lives. There are a number of methods to counter phobias, but apart from living in a bubble with a controlled atmosphere, nothing comes to mind to counter such a phobia.

I have had very bad wind recently. It actually wakes me up at night. I have a healthy diet, with lots of vegetables and whole grains, but could this be a warning of a more serious problem?

Wind is a common symptom and can be difficult to treat. As a general rule, as long as there has not been a change in the frequency of your bowel movements and you are not suffering any pain, excessive mucus, or bleeding from the back passage, it is unlikely that there is a serious cause of your problem. Most people find that having meals that are different from their usual diet will tend to make them produce more wind than usual. This is because the bacteria that live in our bowels get used to coping with whatever we eat on a regular basis, and have a bit more difficulty handling things they're not used to. The gas you are experiencing is produced by the action of bacteria on undigested bowel contents. The amount and type of gas produced in the bowel is therefore directly related to the balance of your diet. One way of reducing the offensive odour from flatulence is to cut down on the amount of meat in the diet.

You may have a mild form of irritable bowel syndrome (IBS), a very common condition causing wind, bloating, crampy abdominal pains and a variable bowel habit. Your doctor can advise you further on this.

Sometimes some anti-spasm medication such as peppermint oil, mebeverine or alverine can help.

Did You Know... The digestive tract is approximately 8 m (30 feet) long in total. Muscles contract in waves to move the food down the oesophagus, meaning that food can get into your stomach even if you are standing on your head.

I have chronic heartburn and it's getting worse. My GP has prescribed me tablets for it but it always comes back when I finish them.

Heartburn conjures up images of overweight and highly stressed businessmen, but stress is not necessarily the cause. Most people will have had heartburn at some time, perhaps after a hot curry. Some people have symptoms just now and then, often related to certain foods, while others have frequent bouts of heartburn that interfere with daily life.

It sounds like you have acid reflux disease, which is more common in smokers, pregnant women, heavy drinkers, the overweight and those aged between 35 and 64. It occurs because your stomach acid leaks or 'refluxes' up into the oesophagus. Inflammation occurs if too much acid remains in contact with the lining of the lower oesophagus, irritating it.

You may have something called a hiatus hernia, where part of the stomach pushes up into the lower part of the chest (above the diaphragm). This can cause reflux, heartburn being the most common symptom.

Tests may be needed if symptoms are severe or not typical. This is to confirm the diagnosis and to rule out other conditions such as heart pains, muscle pains, etc. A common test is a gastroscopy, where a thin, flexible telescope is passed down the oesophagus into the stomach, which allows a doctor to look inside and see if any acid or ulceration is present. Your GP can arrange this for you.

Stop smoking, avoid any foods that seem to make the problem worse and take any tablets with a full glass of water to ensure they are fully swallowed into the stomach. Evening tablets should be taken an hour before bedtime unless otherwise instructed.

The avoidance of hot and spicy foods and ensuring a regular, relatively small dietary intake may also be of benefit.

A useful tip is to raise the head of your bed by 10–15 cm (4–6 inches) to allow gravity to take the acid away from the stomach, and stop it running up into your gullet causing the pain.

Avoid straining during bowel movements, urination and lifting; and avoid tight clothing. Sitting hunched or wearing tight belts puts extra pressure on the stomach, making any reflux worse, so try to avoid this too.

Did You Know... You need a working mouth, oesophagus, stomach, small intestine, large intestine, gallbladder, pancreas and liver just to digest a glass of milk.

Why do I get so bloated?

Bloating, along with variations in the frequency of your bowel movements, are symptoms suggestive of an irritable bowel. It's extremely common, affecting up to one-fifth of us at some time during our lives. The exact causes are not known, but stress and psychological factors may play a significant role.

If you don't have specific food intolerances, then simple dietary advice may help. If bloating is your main symptom, then avoiding too much fibre may help. Intermittent looseness of the stool can be aided with loperamide; and bowel spasm may be helped with mebeverine or Pro-Banthine (propantheline bromide).

We do know that food intolerances such as lactose intolerance may play a part in IBS in a small number of sufferers. Not every person with IBS will have food intolerances, and not every person with food intolerances will have IBS. Try excluding certain food groups from your diet that you think may make your symptoms worse. The most likely culprits are wheat and dairy products. Try two weeks without any dairy products first – if the bloating settles, then you have found out what you need to be cautious about. If it doesn't settle then you can restart the dairy products but cut out wheat for two weeks and see. Make a food diary for a couple of weeks, noting everything you eat and drink and when, and noting your bloating and when it troubles you. You can look over the diary at the end of two weeks to see if you can spot a pattern.

What is the best thing to cure IBS? What's the best diet to go on?

There is no cure for IBS currently, but there are ways of controlling it. The diagnosis is made after taking a medical history and by excluding other possible causes. If investigations for disturbed bowel habit (diarrhoea, constipation, more or less frequent motions), colicky intermittent abdominal pain, bloating and wind are negative, then IBS is the likely diagnosis. There is no specific reliable test for IBS. It is the history of the complaint that points to the diagnosis. The pain of IBS is probably caused by spasm in the bowel, although probably several factors play a part. Some people find that stress makes their symptoms worse. Some women find it is worse at certain times of their menstrual cycle. As both constipation and diarrhoea can occur with IBS, treating the constipation with bulking agents and high-fibre foods can help, but some patients find fibre just makes them feel more bloated and uncomfortable.

Medication can be used to ease the symptoms of IBS, usually antispasmodics, and common ones prescribed are mebeverine, dicyclomine, peppermint oil and alverine.

Did You Know... The average person farts around 14 times each day. You may think that you are far too dignified to eructate, but everyone will at least a few times a day.

I had a serious attack of gastroenteritis four months ago. I was treated with antibiotics but my gut has not been the same since. I am now very sensitive to certain foods and get bloating and diarrhoea. Do I still have the infection?

You have what is known as post-infectious irritable bowel syndrome, where the lining of the bowel is left more sensitive than previously, and which triggers the bowel to go into spasm. This causes a number of symptoms including diarrhoea, constipation, pain and distension but which, fortunately, never goes on to anything more serious. It is extremely common and made worse by stress and certain foods or drinks. It may be sensible to ask your GP to get a stool sample tested for any remaining infection, but I think it is unlikely you will still have one.

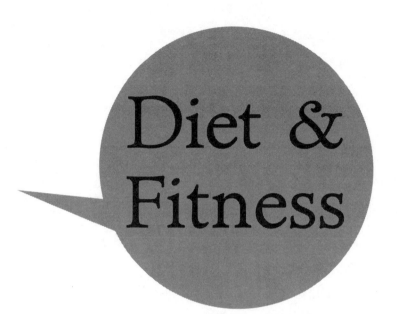

Why should you only eat shellfish when there is an 'R' in the month?

Loads of us love eating shellfish, which include oysters, clams, scallops and mussels, but it is well known that they can make you incredibly sick if you get a dodgy batch. There is some truth in the 'R in the month' rule, and it's all to do with what shellfish eat. Dinoflagellates are a family of single-celled organisms that heavily populate the ocean, floating near the surface, and are the main food group for shellfish. These Dinoflagellates sometimes consume toxic alkaloids called saxitoxins. Because these toxins are more prevalent during May, June, July and August, it is more likely that these toxins will have accumulated in the guts of shellfish caught at this time, which will then get into you when you eat them. Once a shellfish becomes toxic, no amount of heat during cooking will destroy the bacteria. Precautions taken during the raising and harvesting of commercial shellfish make them safe to eat any time of the year, though, so as long as your shellfish has been commercially harvested and is fresh, it should be fine.

Are carrots really good for your eyesight?

Yes and no. Carrots won't improve your vision if you have less than perfect vision, and a diet of carrots won't give a blind person 20/20 vision. But the vitamins found in carrots can help promote overall eye health. Carrots contain beta-carotene, a substance that the body converts to vitamin A, an important nutrient for eye health. A lack of vitamin A can cause blindness. Eat too many carrots, however, and the beta-carotene can turn your skin orange.

Carrots also contain lutein, an antioxidant. Foods rich in lutein have been found to increase pigment density in the macula, the oval-shaped yellow area near the retina of the eye. The greater the pigment density in the macula, the better protected your retina is and the lower your risk of macular degeneration.

Carrots became associated with vision, particularly night vision, during the Second World War when the Royal Air Force published a story that said fighter pilots could thank a steady diet of carrots for their night vision flying prowess. It was, in fact, propaganda put out to conceal the fact that the Royal Air Force was actually using radar to locate Luftwaffe bombers during the night.

Did You Know... 1 in 3 adults and 1 in 5 children is currently obese: that's 13 million obese Britons. The number of overweight people in the world (1,000 million) has overtaken the number of people with not enough to eat (800 million) for the first time.

Why does asparagus make your wee smell?

This has long been the subject of scientific debate and causes much amusement over the dinner table. There are several schools of thought. Some think that people digest asparagus in different ways, being either 'excretors' of the smelly breakdown products, or 'non-excretors'. We also know that not all of us can smell the relevant compounds. Admittedly scientists are still arguing about whether or not all of us produce the chemicals that make the asparagus pee odour, but it certainly seems that, while plenty of people produce it, many can't smell it as they lack the necessary sensory cells in their noses.

The pungent smell is most likely caused by sulphur-containing molecules. One of these, asparagusic acid, is unique to asparagus. It's present in greatest quantities in young plants, and indeed the smell of asparagus pee is most pronounced when you eat young, white asparagus. Another possible compound culprit is called methyl mercaptan, which is the same chemical found in the noxious stink that skunks make. One theory suggests that asparagus breaks down quickly in the body and an enzyme releases methyl mercaptan, which eventually goes through the kidneys and is excreted as a waste product in the urine. Others have blamed chemical compounds called thioesters. It seems the best answer to give you is that we actually don't really know.

Believe it or not, studies have actually been done to investigate this little curiosity, and found that roughly 40 to 50 per cent of those tested developed the distinctive pee smell, and that there is also a proportion of the population who cannot smell the sulphurous fumes of asparagus-laced urine. The studies also suggested that both generating the odoriferous urine and being able to smell it are based on genetics. Only those with a certain gene can break down the chemicals inside the asparagus into their smelly components, and only those with the proper gene can smell the results of that chemical breakdown.

Does spicy food cause ulcers?

Ulcers are essentially sores in the sensitive mucosal lining of the stomach. Ulcers can also occur in the lining of the first section of the small intestine, called the duodenum, or in the oesophagus. You can have more than one ulcer at a time and in more than one place.

For decades doctors believed that eating lots of spicy or highly acidic foods caused ulcers, and so people with ulcers were put on strict, bland diets. This didn't seem to cure the problem, however. It turns out that the vast majority of ulcers are actually caused by a spiral-shaped bacterium called *Helicobacter pylori,* which makes its home in the stomach and duodenum, secreting an enzyme that protects it from the onslaught of stomach acid, and then burrows into the lining, eventually causing an ulcer.

H. pylori is the main cause of ulcers, but not the only cause. Some medications such as aspirin, naproxen and ibuprofen can also irritate the mucosal lining. The risk is greatest in people who take high doses for long periods of time. Spicy food is not to blame.

> **Did You Know...** A normal person has between 25 and 35 billion fat cells, but this number can increase in times of excessive weight gain, to as many as 100 to 150 billion cells.

Is it true that fresh fruits and vegetables are more nutritious than frozen or canned ones?

It depends. Fruit and vegetables that have been languishing in the fridge for a week will probably have lost some of their vitamins – just as they can leach out into cooking water. In that case, 'fresh' produce may not have the same nutritional value as canned or freshly frozen fruits and vegetables. Similarly, if you leave cut-up fresh fruit or vegetables on a kitchen counter for more than 20 minutes, exposure to air may rob them of some of their vitamins. Generally speaking, frozen or canned fruits and vegetables are just as vitamin-rich as fresh.

Which will raise your cholesterol more – beef, poultry or seafood?

How much cholesterol a particular food contains is not the only factor involved in raising your cholesterol. It also depends on the kind of fat the food contains and how this fat affects blood cholesterol levels when eaten. For instance, saturated fat has more of an impact on raising your blood cholesterol levels than the actual cholesterol content of foods, so if the beef is lean and well trimmed, it could contain less cholesterol-boosting saturated fat than a chicken drumstick (dark meat) with the skin on it. Some seafood, such as prawns, may be high in cholesterol but may also contain heart-healthy polyunsaturated fat, which can help lower blood fats.

I have been told to eat dinner early and never to eat after 8 p.m. as it makes you fat. Is this true?

No, there is not an ounce of truth in this. The crackpot theory behind this diet myth is that the body slows down at night and is therefore more prone to gain fat. But there is little evidence that this is anything more than a myth. The same applies to the 'no carbs after 8 p.m.' rule. A calorie is a calorie, whenever you eat it. Eating a large meal just before you go to bed is not a good idea, however, as it can cause indigestion and sleeping problems. But it is your total calorie intake over a 24-hour period balanced against the calories you burn off through your daily activities that matter much more than what time a snack or meal is consumed. What is true is that people who eat late at night tend to go for fattier foods and bigger portions, particularly if they consume their grub in front of the television. This will certainly make them gain weight if they do this regularly.

Did You Know... Some full-fat milk coffee drinks sold in popular coffee-shop chains contain nearly 400 calories – more than 15 per cent of the total (male) daily calorie requirement. A milk-free Americano, by contrast, contains just 17 calories, and a skimmed milk cappuccino around 30.

Why do we need eight glasses of water a day?

The one bit of health 'advice' that I see most often in newspapers and magazines is that we must all be glugging back water, 2 litres or 8 glasses of the stuff a day, but it's simply not true. It's a good way of selling lots of bottles of water, however. Talk to kidney specialists, who know all about matters such as this, and they will tell you that we need around 24ml of fluids per kg in weight each day. If we take in more than this, then we simply excrete it. We do not need to go around clutching bottles of water, either, as any fluids will count, including tea, coffee and juices. We also get a lot of our water from food.

Do certain foods prevent cancer?

Despite many reports that a low-fat diet and plenty of exercise has the potential to prevent cancer, most cancers are down to a question of age, meaning your likelihood of getting cancer increases as you get older. Eating well and exercising will of course contribute to overall wellbeing, and many foods do contain powerful antioxidants that can help to reduce cell damage and the effects of carcinogens, but they should not be viewed as the holy grail of cancer prevention. Many other factors are involved.

Many diets suggest avoiding carbohydrates if you want to lose weight. Is this a good idea?

According to eatwell.gov.uk, the website of the Food Standards Agency, starchy foods only become fattening when actual fat, such as cream or margarine, is added to the meal. Gram for gram, starchy foods contain less than half the calories of fat. Starchy meals should ideally make up a third of the average diet, and the FSA advises using wholegrain varieties where possible, to ensure you receive additional nutrients and fibre. The 'no carbs' fad arose from the Atkins Diet, an unsustainable way of losing weight.

I am 19 and really unhappy with my weight. I can't seem to stick to any of the diets or exercise plans I try. It doesn't seem to matter how much I eat, I never seem to lose any weight. What can I do?

There is no secret to losing weight. It's simple – you need to put fewer calories in your body by eating less or changing the types of food you eat, and burn more calories by exercising. Do that and you will see results. Forget all those ridiculous faddy diets. Eat a healthy, balanced, low-fat diet with plenty of fruit and vegetables. You need to start to make life changes now while you are young and they will become habits for the rest of your life. Join a gym and get exercise advice there, and go to see your doctor to get advice on your diet. Your doctor can also check there are no underlying medical problems that may be causing you to put on weight easily. Start now – you will see the changes quickly and will start feeling much better about yourself.

Did You Know... Women are more likely than men to be obese in all age groups. Babies born to obese mothers may have an increased risk of asthma.

Can you tell me about creatine – is it good to take if you are weight training? And what are the side-effects?

The use of creatine in training for sports remains controversial. Unlike anabolic steroids, which have very well-known and very far-reaching short- and long-term side-effects, creatine remains legal as part of an athlete's training for competition, and its side-effects are generally thought to be much less serious. Certain high-profile celebrities have encouraged many to take creatine, which is generally thought to increase muscle bulk, stamina and performance by up to 10 per cent. It is reported to allow muscle tissue to recover from training and repair itself more quickly. Basically it is the building material for muscle tissue and, because it is rapidly broken down in the body, it seems to feed the muscles more efficiently when taken in synthetic form. But there is a downside; there are certainly side-effects that some people experience, muscle cramps being among the most common. Muscle that grows more quickly may run out of energy supply, making cramps more likely. Since this affects skeletal muscle rather than the muscle in the digestive system, these cramps are particularly likely in the legs and arms.

Should we really not use aluminium pans to cook with anymore – do they cause Alzheimer's?

There is circumstantial evidence linking aluminium with Alzheimer's disease, but no causal relationship has yet been proved. This rumour began a number of years ago when medical researchers found elevated levels of aluminium in the brains of Alzheimer's patients. One possibility was that the raised aluminium level was responsible for causing the disease, and so people started avoiding aluminium cookware – unnecessarily, it turns out. As evidence for other causes continues to grow, this possible link with aluminium seems increasingly unlikely and subsequent research has failed to show any connection between aluminium exposure and Alzheimer's. It is now thought that the elevated aluminium levels found in the brains of Alzheimer's patients is a result of the disease process itself, not the other way round. In other words, high aluminium levels do not cause Alzheimer's, but rather Alzheimer's causes high aluminium levels.

Do diet cola drinks damage your bones?

Research has confirmed that regularly drinking cola – including diet varieties – is bad for women's bones and may increase the risk of osteoporosis in later life. It's most likely due to the high levels of phosphoric acid in the cola interfering with bone formation. As part of the normal ageing process, bones lose calcium more quickly than it can be replaced, leading to a reduction in bone density. As a result, the bones gradually lose their strength and become more brittle. The National Osteoporosis Society recommends cutting down on fizzy drinks to keep bones strong, not just because phosphoric acid has the potential to weaken bones but also because too much caffeine affects the balance of calcium in the body, too.

Did You Know... Obesity and being overweight pose a major risk for chronic diseases, including type 2 diabetes, cardiovascular disease, hypertension and stroke, and certain forms of cancer.

Do men lose weight faster than women?

A 16-month study looking at the effects of exercising on weight loss involved men and women completing an identical amount of exercise each week. The results showed that, on average, men lost 5 kg (11 lb) while women lost nothing. Unfair, isn't it? Why did this happen? One theory is that it may be due to an evolutionary effect designed to protect women's role as child-bearers, ensuring that they maintain adequate body fat for nourishing healthy babies. Hence women are much more energy-efficient and lose less weight. Sorry, ladies.

Will drinking lots of water help me to lose weight?

Well, actually it may do – provided that the water is cold. Drinking at least eight glasses of ice-cold water a day can help you to lose weight. Not only does water suppress your appetite by making the stomach feel fuller, but it also lowers your body temperature, causing your metabolism to rise to try to produce more heat. If you don't drink enough your kidneys can't do their job properly, and so your liver is required to do much of their job. This means that it is not so involved in burning fat, so some of the fat that would normally be used as fuel gets stored in your body instead. Keeping well-hydrated means your liver can concentrate on metabolizing fat.

My friend told me to put lemon juice on my food as it dissolves fat. Is this true?

Although it's a good source of vitamin C, it won't dissolve the fat in fatty foods. It might just dissolve your teeth, however, due to the high acidity of the juice. There is no way of cutting fat from your food other than physically removing it yourself, or taking certain medications which block the absorption of fat in your intestines.

I never eat breakfast but still have a weight problem – and it is getting worse! Why?

People who miss breakfast are more likely to put on weight, according to a number of researchers. A study looking at lifestyle differences and weight trends in more than 35,000 adolescents showed that those who skipped breakfast were 2.2 times more likely to be overweight. In fact, the single most important risk factor for being overweight and obese was skipping breakfast. A study done at Harvard Medical School of 6,000 men found that among those who ate breakfast the risk of putting on weight was reduced by a quarter.

Low-fat meals mean low-calorie meals, right?

A common misconception is that low-fat and fat-free foods are also low in calories. Actually, many processed low-fat or fat-free foods have as many – or in some cases more – calories than full-fat foods because they have more sugar and other high-calorie compounds added to improve flavour and texture (both of which can deteriorate when fat is removed). So if you're trying to lose weight, remember to check the calorie content of even low-fat foods.

I can remember being told that you burn more calories eating celery than you actually get from it. Are there really fat-burning foods like this, or is it a myth?

Claims that celery and some other foods can 'burn' calories are not backed up by any research. No foods can 'burn' fat, and it's a myth about celery. Some foods with caffeine may speed up your metabolism for a short time, but they do not cause weight loss. Taking in fewer calories and burning more through activity will help you lose weight.

Did You Know... Obesity increases the chances of developing osteoarthritis. This is because the excess body weight puts more stress on the joint cartilage.

I want to go to the gym to lose weight and my trainer says I should do weights, but won't this make me bulky?

Many women are put off weight-lifting as an exercise to lose weight because they worry that they will bulk up. But lifting weights and doing push-ups and crunches regularly can help with weight loss. The more fit and toned your muscles are, the more efficiently they burn calories, even at rest. Exercising two to three days a week will not lead to bulking up. Only intense strength training, combined with a certain genetic background, will build very large muscles.

Why do I always end up putting more weight on after I've been on my summer bikini diet?

Cutting out too many calories too quickly can be disastrous. You will lose weight at the start, but then your metabolism slows down to adapt to the lower calorie intake, allowing your body to function with less fuel. This means that nearly every calorie that you eat will be carefully conserved and stored as fat. This is why people who go on extreme diets pile the pounds back on as soon as they start eating normally again. When calories are cut too low, it is mostly water rather than fat that is lost, and the body starts breaking down its own muscle protein for fuel, slowing the metabolism even further.

Top 10 Toxic But Everyday Foods

1) Pufferfish

This one is well known. It's the second most poisonous vertebrate in the world, yet some parts of the fish are considered to be delicacies. The poison in the fish, known as *tetrodotoxin*, can cause numbness, high blood pressure and muscle paralysis, which leads to death as the diaphragm muscles become paralysed. Interestingly, it is illegal for the Emperor of Japan to eat pufferfish.

2) Cassava

Hugely popular in the Caribbean, South America and Africa, cassava is a dietary staple for millions. Yet its taste and smell depend on the amount of cyanogenic glucosides it contains, which are, in fact, extremely poisonous. If cassava is prepared incorrectly, it can be deadly due to high levels of cyanide, which cause irreversible paralysis.

Cassava roots are ground into flour, which is used to make tapioca. The deadly cyanide is broken down if the flour is left in the shade for five hours.

3) Mushrooms

There are 38,000 known types of mushrooms, but relatively few are actually toxic: only around 5 per cent, in fact. One of the deadliest types of mushroom toxins is *alpha-amanitin*, which causes extreme liver damage. Toadstools, as they are called, are the most poisonous.

4) Chillies

Everyone has eaten a chilli or two, and whether it was scorching hot or extremely mild it would have contained a chemical called *capsaicin*. It's this that gives them their fiery heat. Eat enough capsaicin and it can kill you. The chemical is so strong that it is used as a paint stripper and in the pepper spray used by police forces. Very strong chillies can actually burn the skin during preparation and handling.

5) Cashews

Misnamed a nut, the cashew is actually a seed that grows inside a shell-like structure on a fruit. You can't buy truly raw cashews, as they contain urushiol, the same chemical found in poison ivy, and so can cause a similar reaction. If large amounts are eaten, it can be deadly. Poisoning is rare, but workers who handle them to get the shells off can sometimes experience the adverse effects. In South American countries the fruit of the cashew is eaten and the seed (the bit we eat) is thrown away.

6) Potatoes

Most gardeners will know, but not many members of the general public, that potatoes are in fact toxic. The stem and leaves of the plant and even the potato itself are toxic. Their raw greenish colour is due to levels of glycoalkaloid poison, which has caused some deaths in the past. And this death doesn't come suddenly, either. It usually results in gradual weakness and then a coma. Avoid any green bits and cook all potatoes properly.

7) Almonds

Like cashews, almonds are also actually seeds. They are also extremely poisonous if not introduced to some sort of heat source. It is generally the bitter almonds that need treating to get rid of the poison, as they are full of cyanide. In many countries it is illegal to sell them without having processed the poison out first.

8) Cherries

This may come as a surprise. Cherries can be eaten raw, cooked, baked and made either tart or sweet. But despite their appeal and versatility, cherries are toxic. Chew the stone and you are likely to introduce cyanide into your body, as any damage to the stones automatically produces hydrogen cyanide. Symptoms of mild poisoning include headache, dizziness, confusion, anxiety and vomiting, while larger doses can lead to difficulty breathing, increased blood pressure and heart rate, and kidney failure. Reactions can include coma, convulsions, and death from respiratory arrest.

9) Apples
Popular everywhere, like many other types of fruits apples do actually contain low levels of cyanide. Not in the fruit itself, but in the seeds. Eating all of the seeds in one apple won't kill you, but it's definitely not to be recommended.

10) Tomatoes
It's true, they really are poisonous. The stem as well as the leaves contains a chemical known as *glycoalkaloid*, a chemical known to cause upset stomachs and nervousness. Higher levels are found in wild tomatoes, but those grown domestically still contain glycoalkaloid. This chemical is so powerful that it is also used as a way to control pests.

Which is the best fad/celebrity diet?

There isn't one. The cabbage soup diet, the low-carbohydrate diet, etc. all promise to fight fat and shrink stomachs. But they are not recommended for losing weight. Fad diets usually overemphasize one particular food or type of food, contradicting the guidelines for good nutrition. They may work at first because they cut calories, but they rarely have a permanent effect.

I don't think that it is my fault that I'm fat. It's all to do with my genes, isn't it?

Recent studies have shown that our genes can indeed influence obesity. People who inherit one version of a gene called FTO are 70 per cent more likely to be obese than those who inherit another. And there are seven more genetic regions that influence body weight. However, of the seven variants identified, five are active in the brain. The implication is that they affect obesity not by changing people's metabolisms, but their behaviour. For example, you may have a gene that increases appetite. In that case, we cannot lazily blame DNA for an expanding waistline. There is nothing in our biology to stop us from losing weight if we consume fewer calories and join a gym. The task might be harder for people with one genetic profile than another, but no gene compels us to have second helpings.

Did You Know... Child and adolescent obesity is also associated with increased risk of emotional problems. Teens with weight problems tend to have much lower self-esteem and be less popular with their peers.

I see these 'flex' products on the market that use small electric currents to tone your muscles. Are these products dangerous to use, and do they actually work?

These products make your muscles contract using an electric current. They are very safe and work exactly the same way as the TENS units used to ease pain in childbirth. The current used is very small. There is no evidence that the current used has any bad effects whatsoever. There really is no substitute for proper physical exercise, however, as the stimulation of muscles you get from exercise is very many times greater and more effective than when the muscles are being exercised passively. These machines do nothing to raise the heart or respiratory rate, and therefore have no effect whatsoever in improving cardiovascular fitness, which is the aspect of exercise that does you most good.

What's the best way to detox?

The word 'detox' has become the bane of my life. It represents a multi-million-pound industry and has spawned so much pseudo-science on packaging, boxes and in magazines that it has become an established term, despite being devoid of all meaning or scientific sense. It's a hugely successful marketing gimmick that has persuaded apparently intelligent men and women to part with large sums of money for colonic treatments and post-partying cleansing rituals that are about as effective as a chocolate teapot.

There is no such thing as 'detoxing'. Your body comes with several remarkably efficient organs that can remove most harmful substances from your body: your liver and your kidneys. If human beings stored toxins as much as the manufacturers of detox products would have you believe, then we would have died out years ago.

Gentle exercise and adequate fluids are all that are needed to get the human body back on track after a period of over-indulgence. Anything else (colonics included) is a waste of time and money.

What exactly are probiotics and these 'friendly bacteria' that are always being advertised? Do they do us any good or is it just marketing?

The smooth and efficient functioning of your gut depends on having a certain amount and types of bacteria in the intestines to help break down food. Since antibiotics, alcohol, stress, pollutants and processed foods can all reduce the level of these 'friendly bacteria', the theory is that you should take probiotics to replace them.

Common probiotics include various species of the bacteria *Bifidobacterium* and *Lactobacillus*. Much research has actually been done on them and the US government's lead agency for scientific research on complementary and alternative medicine and the American Society for Microbiology have concluded that these bacteria may be helpful to treat diarrhoea, infections of the urinary tract or female genital tract, irritable bowel syndrome and some intestinal infections.

An analysis published in the *Canadian Medical Association Journal* of six studies involving 836 children on antibiotics showed that those who also took a probiotic had far less diarrhoea than those who took just the antibiotic.

The problem lies in the quality of the many probiotic products available. Research suggests that half of the available products either do not contain the right bacteria or do not contain enough to have any effect.

There was an old treatment used for patients who had developed a certain type of diarrhoea while on strong antibiotics in hospital – the poo enema. While it sounds revolting, the thought behind it is actually quite brilliant. In these patients their antibiotic treatment had wiped out all their normal bugs, allowing diarrhoeal ones to grow. If you squirt a solution of someone else's poo up the bottom, the good bacteria in the poo will re-colonize the gut and so compete with the bad bugs, killing them. Quite brilliantly simple and remarkably effective – although the patients didn't always see it that way!

Did You Know... The largest internal organ is the small intestine. Despite being called the smaller of the two intestines, your small intestine is actually four times as long as the average adult is tall. If it weren't looped back and forth upon itself, it wouldn't fit inside the abdominal cavity.

I have developed lactose intolerance. Is avoiding milk the only solution? Should I try desensitization or something? If I drink only a small amount nothing bad happens.

If you have lactose intolerance, then the only thing to do at present is to avoid milk and all dairy products that contain lactose. It is not possible to desensitize yourself to the lactose. However, if you follow a strict regime for a year or so and you have no problems, it can be worthwhile trying at that stage to slowly reintroduce lactose products, as the intolerance may occasionally go away and not be life-long.

For the moment, though, it is best to avoid dairy products altogether.

I am a teenager and I want to start lifting weights to get a bit bigger for rugby, but everyone is saying that it will stunt my growth. Is this actually true?

Everyone used to say this when I was at school. It was a great excuse to stay out of the gym and avoid PE! But it's not at all true. The whole notion of growth being stunted by weight-lifting is a myth. There is living proof: Arnold Schwarzenegger started weight-lifting very young and is 6 ft 1in, and Lou Ferrigno of *The Incredible Hulk* started working out at 14 years old and is now 6 ft 5 in. Weight-lifting does not stunt height growth, or any other kind of growth, for that matter. There is no scientific evidence to support such ideas and, in fact, books such as *The Russian School of Height* suggest that weight-training may stimulate growth. The latest weight-training studies done on teens showed only positive effects – so long as the training is done correctly. It's interesting to note that running and jumping can create forces on the body that are six to eight times one's body weight. This means that the compression forces on your legs and spine are far greater when you are running and jumping than they will ever be doing squats or bench presses.

If the idea of aerobic exercise is to get your heart pumping at an accelerated rate for a sustained period, then why can't you get a good workout by drinking large amounts of coffee? How come it's good when aerobics makes your heart pound faster, but bad when coffee does the same thing?

Ha, you are trying to be clever, aren't you? The problem is you are focusing only on the parts, rather than the whole. The key to aerobics is not just to get the heart pumping faster, but also to get the entire complex of heart, lungs, muscles, blood and blood vessels operating with maximum efficiency. Although heart rate is often assessed during a workout, it's not really a good measure of how hard you are working. That would come from measuring oxygen consumption.

Merely getting your heart pounding from caffeine will not have anywhere near the same effect, and may well raise your blood pressure and cause heart arrhythmias and other undesirable things.

You could ask a similar question: isn't a fat person who loses a lot of weight better off than a person who's been skinny all his life, because the fat person has been doing years of involuntary weight-lifting carrying his own heavy body around? But this is not true, either, because as obesity increases, activity decreases. The obese may be carting around a lot more weight than average, but they move a lot less than average, too.

So I'm afraid you still need to hit the gym, not the coffee shop.

Did You Know... The skin represents 12–16 per cent of a body's total weight!

Is spinach as high in iron as Popeye and my mother say?

Everyone thinks of spinach as a good source of iron almost exclusively because of Popeye. But it's a myth. It arose from a typing error in which the decimal point was put in the wrong place. This gave spinach the reputation of having 10 times more iron then any other green leafy vegetable. It doesn't. The creator of the Popeye comic strip had read this erroneous piece of info and decided to use it, thereby securing it in the minds of the public for the last 60 years.

In fact, spinach has a drawback: even though it contains high levels of iron and calcium, the rate of absorption is almost nil as it also contains oxalic acid, which binds calcium and iron, blocking their absorption. So while spinach is a rich source of vitamin A, vitamin E, beta carotene and several vital antioxidants, it's actually a poor source of iron.

It is never a good idea to rely on a single food group as a source of a particular nutrient. Instead, it's far better to eat a wide range of foods.

I love to go to the steam room and sauna after a workout. But I've always wondered: Do they really help? What exactly are the benefits – or am I actually damaging my body?

The truth is, we don't really know. What little research there is has given very mixed results. One American study claimed that very few sudden deaths take place during or after a sauna, but a Finnish study found that almost all (221 of 228) hyperthermia deaths in Finland from 1970 to 1986 took place in saunas. It should be mentioned that most of the overheated dead were middle-aged men under the influence of alcohol.

Saunas can help people with chronic heart failure, asthma or chronic bronchitis; they reduce pain and increase mobility in people with arthritis, and enhance resistance to the common cold. They also decrease lung congestion and seem to lower blood pressure in those with hypertension. But they are a bad idea during a high-risk pregnancy, and are also contraindicated for various cardiac conditions other than chronic heart failure.

Perhaps the best advice I can give you is that if you're in good health, a sauna or steam bath won't kill you, and possibly may help you catch fewer colds.

Did You Know... You use 200 muscles to take one step. That's a lot of work for the muscles, considering most of us take about 10,000 steps a day.

Are artificial sweeteners safe or do they cause cancer?

The main sweetener involved in this heated debate is aspartame. A lot of studies have recommended further investigation into the possible connection between aspartame and diseases such as brain tumours and lymphoma. There was also much controversy around some alleged conflicts of interest in the approval process, and these have fuelled the fire.

Aspartame is broken down into aspartic acid by the body. Because the additive aspartame is metabolized and absorbed very quickly, it can cause very high levels of aspartic acid in the blood. This does not occur with natural sources of aspartame.

Aspartic acid belongs to a class of chemicals that can act as 'excitotoxins', which damage brain cells and nerve cells. Aspartic acid does not normally cross the blood–brain barrier in most parts of the brain, but high levels of excitotoxins have been shown (in hundreds of studies on animals) to cause damage to areas of the brain unprotected by the blood–brain barrier.

Some scientists think that aspartame may affect neuro-transmitter production, and that even a moderate increase in levels of aspartame in the blood plasma – as can result from taking in a typical amount – may have adverse consequences with long-term use.

A professor of clinical psychiatry surveyed 166 studies of aspartame in peer-reviewed medical literature and found that 74 studies had Nutrasweet industry-related funding, while 92 were independently funded. All of the industry-funded research found aspartame to be safe, whereas 92 per cent of the independently funded research identified a problem with it. Hmmmmmm…

It's been reported that complaints about aspartame make up 75 per cent of all reports of adverse reactions to substances in the food supply, and a total of 92 different symptoms and health conditions have been reported.

In 1992 the US Air Force issued an alert warning its pilots about drinking diet drinks containing aspartame before flying.

It does make you wonder.

Does cheese really give you bad dreams?

Nearly every parent is guilty of warning their children not to eat cheese before going to bed because it will give them bad dreams. But this is not based on any sound science whatsoever. In fact, researchers have found that cheese can actually aid sleep. Volunteers were fed a 20g piece of cheese every night before going to sleep: 72 per cent slept very well, and 70 per cent remembered their dreams, none of which was a nightmare.

While it doesn't cause bad dreams, the *type* of cheese you choose *can* affect the dreams you have: Stilton causes the craziest dreams, Cheddar-eaters have more dreams about celebrities, and nostalgic dreams of old friends and the past seem to be prompted by eating Red Leicester. Cheshire cheese seems to induce the best night's sleep of all, with over half of the volunteers reporting completely dreamless sleep.

I'm not really sure where the cheese and nightmares myth originated. Charles Dickens' character Ebenezer Scrooge blames 'a crumb of cheese' for his night-time visitations in *A Christmas Carol*, and a health scare in the 1950s found cheese to be problematic for people using a particular antidepressant. But that's all I can come up with.

What actually happens when you get a 'stitch' in your side during exercise?

The pain you feel when you have a 'stitch' is most likely emanating from muscles or ligaments somewhere in the region of the abdomen. Some think it's caused by a muscle spasm of the diaphragm, but it could also be cramping or straining of the ligaments in the diaphragm/liver area. Someone clearly thought about this a great deal and suggested that runners who breathe out when their right foot strikes the ground put more pressure on the right side, where the diaphragm is located, and will therefore be more prone to getting stitches.

Taking deep breaths, exhaling forcefully while running hard and paying special attention to which foot you land on as you breathe out can all help to reduce stitches.

Did You Know... The tooth is the only part of the human body that can't repair itself. The outer layer of the tooth is enamel, which is not living tissue so it can't self-repair.

I always left the crusts of bread as a child but my parents said that these were the healthiest bit and I should eat them. Surely bread is all the same, all over?

Loads of kids leave their crusts, but there is actually a crumb of truth (sorry) in your parents' advice. A study published in the American Chemical Society's *Journal of Agricultural and Food Chemistry* showed that bread crusts not only contain a powerful concentration of antioxidants, which may help to reduce the risk of some cancers, but also are also rich in dietary fibre, which can prevent colon cancer.

When bread is baked, the heat causes carbon found in the carbohydrates of the bread to combine with the amino acids of the proteins, resulting in a browning of the surface of the bread. This process is known as the Maillard reaction, discovered by Louis-Camille Maillard in the early 1900s. Researchers have now shown that the Maillard reaction produces the many antioxidants found in bread crusts.

Similar research from Germany experimented with an everyday sourdough bread mixture. By analysing the bread crust, bread crumbs from the paler inside of the bread and raw flour, the researchers discovered that pronyl-lysine, an important antioxidant, was eight times more plentiful in the bread crust than in other parts of the loaf. Interestingly, pronyl-lysine was not present in the flour at all. So eating the crusts does have its benefits, and if you're a parent you should encourage your kids to do so!

My cholesterol level is high. My diet is generally good but I want to know what you think of Benecol (the cholesterol-reducing spread)? Does it work?

A lot of research has been done into these cholesterol-lowering dietary additives, and several have been found that do indeed work. Many are natural substances that reduce the absorption of cholesterol from the gut and so lower cholesterol levels in the blood.

A 2g average daily portion of these substances added to margarine can reduce the average LDL cholesterol level by between 0.3 and 0.5 mmol/l, reducing your risk of heart disease by as much as 25 per cent.

But remember that cholesterol levels alone aren't the whole story. It is the *type* of cholesterol (LDL = bad, HDL = good) and the presence of other risk factors for cardiovascular disease that determine the significance of any particular cholesterol level. Even in someone with a healthy lifestyle, the cholesterol profile sometimes remains so unfriendly that it raises risk to an unacceptable level. Occasionally it is necessary to use prescription medication to lower cholesterol.

Why does eating chocolate make me so happy? If it didn't I wouldn't be fat!

Chocolate is a natural mood-enhancer because it contains a substance called phenylethylamine, which belongs to the group of chemicals known as endorphins. They have a stimulating effect on the brain, causing a sense of happiness and wellbeing as well as an increase in positive energy. Phenylethylamine is also found in cheese and certain kinds of sausages, but unfortunately neither of these makes a particularly satisfactory or healthy chocolate substitute.

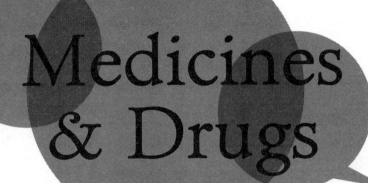

Medicines & Drugs

I am very overweight and haven't had much luck with dieting. What prescription medicines are available to help me?

Fortunately, dieting is not actually about luck but is about choosing and sticking to a sensible eating plan. There is currently one main weight-loss drug available, but it is prescribed only if certain criteria are met. It's called Xenical, and it works by blocking the absorption of about 30 per cent of the fat you eat, causing it to pass straight through. This can help boost weight-loss efforts when used with a program of healthy eating and exercise. It does have some pretty nasty side-effects if you don't stick to a sensible diet – eat high-fat foods and you will experience bloating, flatulence and even faecal incontinence of very oily stools.

Can you tell me about a pill you can take to stop smoking?

Giving up smoking can be very hard but is well worth the effort, as it is the single biggest preventable cause of disease and premature death. Smokers have double the risk of heart diseases compared to non-smokers. The drug bupropion (Zyban) was developed as an antidepressant but can work to help smokers quit. You start taking one tablet a day one week before stopping smoking and continue for two months. Nicotine patches or gum can be used at the same time. The drug's main side-effect is sleep disturbance and dry mouth. You can get it from your NHS GP. There is another medication called varenicline (Champix) that also acts on the brain to help you stop smoking. It should be started one to two weeks before you quit, and is taken twice a day.

Did You Know... There are over 4,000 dangerous chemicals in cigarette, cigar and pipe smoke. Many of these chemicals are cancer-causing.

Why can't you drink alcohol if you are taking antibiotics?

This is actually a big misconception. Drinking alcohol while on antibiotics will not hinder their efficacy in any way. There are only two antibiotics that can react with alcohol, resulting in nasty side-effects: metronidazole and tinidazole. Drinking when taking these can cause flushing, headaches and vomiting. A glass of wine or two when taking penicillin is not going to cause you any problems.

Could you please tell me something about Viagra and other pills such as Kamagra? How safe are they? Will herbal Viagra work instead?

Viagra is something of a cult drug now, but caused a lot of controversy when it first came out. It is used for erection problems and can also help with premature ejaculation. You take it only when you want to have sex. It works by increasing blood flow to the penis. Normally, erection is achieved because when a man is sexually stimulated, the arteries in the penis relax and enlarge. As these arteries expand the veins taking blood away from the penis are compressed, restricting the blood flow out of the penis and causing an erection. If the nerves and blood vessels that facilitate this process are not working sufficiently, then erection problems occur. Effects from Viagra can be noticed in a short time and can last for up to four hours. Contrary to popular belief it will only give you an erection if you are aroused – you won't have one all the time.

Kamagra is basically the same thing – a sort of Viagra copy. It contains exactly the same drug, but I would imagine that the quality and quantity of drug in the tablets is variable, as any company can make Kamagra. Given the choice I would opt for genuine Viagra obtained from a doctor.

Herbal Viagra is not something I can recommend. Erectile problems should always be checked out by a doctor, as they can be a sign of a more serious underlying problem such as heart disease or diabetes.

I am a 45-year-old male with high blood pressure, treated with beta-blockers. My problem is that I am now impotent. Is it my blood pressure pills that are causing it?

Impotence (erectile dysfunction) is a well-known side-effect of beta-blockers and so it would not be unreasonable to ask your GP to try a different blood pressure tablet to see if things improve down below. With the exception of 'thiazide diuretics', sexual difficulties are less likely with other forms of blood pressure treatment. Most doctors (and patients) would regard erectile dysfunction as an unacceptable side-effect and are very ready to suggest other options. Possible options for you may be calcium channel blockers, ACE inhibitors, angiotensin-2 receptor antagonists and alpha-blockers.

Did You Know... An estimated 1.3 billion people are smokers worldwide. Smoking is set to kill 6.5 million people in 2015 and 8.3 million humans in 2030, with the biggest rise in low- and middle-income countries. Tobacco use will kill 1 billion people in the 21st century if current smoking trends continue.

Are cigars better for you than cigarettes, or are they just as bad for your health?

Many people give up cigarettes only to start smoking cigars as a replacement. Or the argument goes that one doesn't inhale cigars, and therefore they pose no health risks. However, this couldn't be further from the truth. Concentrations of tar and nicotine are much higher in cigars than cigarettes. Cigar smoke is also more likely to cause persistent coughs and phlegm, as well as an increased risk of peptic ulcers.

It is also worth noting that a cigar can produce over 20 times as much second-hand smoke as a cigarette. That's more than enough for all the family to enjoy. The bottom line is that cancer death rates for cigar smokers are over 30 per cent higher than for non-smokers. With this kind of statistic it really is immaterial whether cigars or cigarettes are healthier: they are both killers. End of story.

Can eating poppy seeds make you fail a drugs test?

This is something often debated at dinner parties, and plays on the fact that we are all afraid of random drug testing. We may be against it, but we all want our pilots to be clean and sober.

Random drug screenings tend to use urine, and work by using antibodies directed at the compound the test is looking for. In the case of an opiate test they are looking for codeine and morphine in the urine, the two substances that heroin is broken down into. Poppy seeds do actually contain codeine and morphine, but in a very low concentration. Studies have shown that a person can test positive for up to 72 hours after eating a poppy seed bagel. Many of these tests are highly sensitive and can detect as little as 300 nanograms (that's one-billionth of a gram) of codeine, so yes, eating poppy seeds can make you fail a drugs test.

Many people have said that lip balms contain ingredients that make chapped lips worse, to keep you using them and buying more, but I can't believe that the manufacturers could get away with that. Is it true?

Incredibly, this is partly true. The ingredients of lip balms often include substances that cause a tingling, such as salicylic acid, phenol and menthol. These ingredients are routinely used to make the consumer think something is happening when they apply the balm. Some of these are exfoliants that cause the lips to peel. This then makes the lips become thinner and less able to protect against the elements, so people keep applying the balm. Many people have experienced chapped lips despite diligently applying 'medicated' lip balm several times a day.

Camphor and menthol are known as counter-irritants, and dry out the lips – a necessary step for healing cold sores, but too extreme for ordinary dryness. Phenol's main purpose is to kill bacteria and help prevent infections, and should be used only in severe cases, not on a daily basis. Users, meanwhile, often find the pleasant tingling habit-forming.

Would a dermatologist prescribe salicylic acid for chapped lips? It's very unlikely, as it is a peeling agent, so it would help cold sores, but chapped lips need a lubricant (like petroleum jelly/ Vaseline), not an exfoliant.

Top 10 Curious Allergies

1) Nickel

I am one of around 1 per cent of the population that has a nickel allergy. It's certainly not rare, but has become more widely known as the use of technology has increased and users of mobile phones, MP3 players, etc. notice that the nickel contained in the casings irritates them. Many everyday items contain it, including coins, jewellery, studs in clothing, scissors, kitchen utensils, and even chairs.

2) Caffeine

Intolerance to caffeine is a pretty common ailment, but there are people for whom ingesting even the smallest amount can lead to a life-threatening allergic reaction. Those allergic to caffeine can experience delusions, anxiety attacks, hallucinations, muscle jerks, rashes, hives, heart palpitations and blurry vision. Some even experience fatal seizures.

3) Wood

Strange but true. Some people are allergic to certain types of wood or sawdust, others are allergic to any type of wood in many forms, whether it is dust or solid. This means that they can't touch paper or use a pencil or wooden-handled tools. The allergy can be so strong that it can cause the skin to look as if it has been burned.

4) Plastic

Plastics are everywhere, so this allergy can be particularly trying. It means no drinking from water bottles, no food storage boxes, certain types of glasses can't be worn, no credit cards or even plastic utensils. Sufferers can experience skin irritations such as a rash, swelling, redness and itching.

5) Electromagnetic Hypersensitivity

Allergies to technology like computers and mobile phones may seem highly unlikely today, but sufferers complain of nasal congestion, sneezing, itching and even headaches after using computers. Research has found that computer monitors and other parts contain a chemical called triphenyl phosphate, which is used as a flame retardant. It is this that seems to be responsible for the discomfort of these sufferers.

6) Kissing

Well, OK, this isn't strictly an allergy simply to kissing. People who suffer from this allergy usually have a severe food or medicinal allergy that can be triggered through kissing by the close contact and sharing of saliva, food particles or particles from medicine left in the mouth.

7) Exercise

Very often this is simply an excuse not to work out, but around 1,000 people are thought to have this allergy. Called exercise-induced anaphylaxis, it's usually only noticed after someone eats a certain type of food, say, peanuts, and goes to exercise. That person can easily eat peanuts without having a reaction, but when exercise is added, the person may experience fainting, vomiting and difficulty breathing.

8) Cold

Not many of us love the cold weather, but some are actually allergic to it. Also called Familial Cold Auto-inflammatory Syndrome, cold weather can trigger the body to release histamine in the skin, which causes rashes, hives, redness and swelling. It can be deadly if undiagnosed, especially if the affected person jumps into a cold pool or has a cold shower, which may cause the body to go into shock.

9) Sun

Erythropoietic protoporphyria is the more complex name, and while it is extremely rare, it does exist. It is thought that only 300 people in the world are allergic to the sun. When exposed to direct sunlight, the immune system activates inflammatory cells within the skin that cause damage. Sufferers need to wear special clothing and avoid the sun at all costs.

10) Water

The correct medical term is aquagenic urticaria, and it affects one in 23 million people in the world. Most are confined to their homes, and being allergic to water means also being allergic to sweat, tears and even foods that contain water such as juices, tea and coffee. Bathing and showering are obviously extremely difficult. The cause seems to be a hypersensitivity to the ions found in non-distilled water, so most have to drink distilled water.

Can breathalysers be fooled by putting something in your mouth before the test?

It's sad to think that so many people have spent so many hours trying to work out how to fool alcohol breathalysers instead of just not drink-driving. Breath mints, mouthwash and onion have all been tried and found to be ineffective. Adding an odour to mask the smell of alcohol might fool a person, but doesn't change the actual alcohol concentration in the body or on the breath.

Products such as mouthwash or breath spray can actually 'fool' breath machines by significantly raising test results. Listerine, for example, contains 27 per cent alcohol and will result in a falsely high test reading. Because of this, most instruments require that the individual be tested twice at least two minutes apart. Mouthwash or other mouth alcohol will have dissipated after two minutes and cause the second reading to disagree with the first, requiring a retest.

For the sake of giving you a complete answer, there are substances that might actually reduce blood alcohol readings. These include a bag of activated charcoal concealed in the mouth (to absorb alcohol vapour), an oxidizing gas (such as N_2O, C_{12}, O_3, etc.) that would fool a fuel-cell type detector, or an organic interferent to fool an infra-red absorption detector. Fortunately these are not at all practical to apply, and difficult to get hold of. Best just not drink, eh?

Did You Know... Each day 3,000 children smoke their first cigarette.

Do some nasal sprays actually make congestion and runny noses worse?

Yes. Nasal sprays work by decreasing the flow of blood to the lining of the nose, so the tissue becomes less congested and mucous production is slowed. Frequent use of these decongestants, however (for example oxymetazoline, phenylephrine and xylometazoline nasal sprays, which work by constricting the blood vessels in the lining of the nose), can cause rebound nasal congestion. This typically occurs after 5 to 7 days of regular use of such medications. One study has shown that the anti-infection agent benzalkonium chloride, which is frequently added to nasal sprays, aggravates the condition further. Patients often try increasing both the dose and the frequency of use of the nasal spray when this happens, in an attempt to treat it. The swelling of the nasal passages caused by rebound congestion may eventually result in a condition called permanent turbinate hyperplasia, which may block breathing through the nose completely until the blockage is removed surgically.

The treatment is to stop using the offending nasal spray. Either a 'cold turkey' or a 'weaning' approach can be used. Symptoms of congestion and runny nose can often be relieved by using prescription nasal steroid sprays one to two times daily for a few weeks. For very severe cases, oral steroids may be necessary. Oral decongestant medications like pseudoephedrine can also help while you're switching away from over-the-counter nasal spray.

Do truth serums really exist?

Pliny the Elder coined the phrase *in vino veritas* ('in wine, truth') and thereby described the first and oldest truth serum. He was basically saying that anything that lowers your inhibitions is likely to cause you to spill the beans.

The earliest confession induced using something stronger than wine was reported in 1903 when a New York cop admitted under the influence of ether that he'd faked insanity when accused of killing his wife.

The first drug to really start being used as a truth serum was scopolamine. Mixed with morphine, it was used from the 1940s to the 1960s to help women in labour forget the pain (they still experienced it, mind!). A Texan obstetrician claimed his patients always answered truthfully when under its influence – the drug targets areas of the brain to do with self-control – and the age of truth serum investigation was born.

Scopolamine was soon abandoned in favour of safer drugs such as sodium amytal and sodium thiopental.

The problem with truth serums is that the results can't be depended on. Also, just because a person under the influence of a truth serum believes something to be true, that doesn't mean it actually is.

The US Supreme Court has now ruled that confessions obtained using drugs are inadmissible as evidence, as has the European Court of Human Rights.

Is 'roid rage real? Nobody seems to question whether steroid rage actually exists but isn't it just bodybuilder myth?

The steroids that bodybuilders use are synthetic hormones that are administered in high doses to produce an exaggerated version of the physiological changes caused by natural hormones. The most obvious physical effect of these artificial male sex hormones is an increase in muscle size, but one common psychological effect is increased aggressiveness, known, as in your question, as 'roid rage. It does indeed happen, but not to everybody. Most steroid users experience little or no psychological effect at all.

It's worth mentioning that women aren't immune to such effects, either. A study of 75 women athletes found that one-third used steroids and, of that third, more than half suffered from irritability, and 40 per cent reported an increase in aggressive behaviour.

Plenty of research has linked steroid use to violence and crime. A Swedish study of male prison inmates found those testing positive for steroids were more than twice as likely as non-users to have committed weapons offences, and a study of 12- to 17-year-olds found that those who had used steroids at least once had committed criminal property damage at twice the rate of non-users.

Did You Know... Humans shed about 600,000 particles of skin every hour, and regrow outer skin cells about every 27 days. Chances are that last month's skin is still hanging around your house in the form of 'dust'.

Why does grapefruit so often appear on lists of things you mustn't mix with certain medicines?

Grapefruit juice and the fruit itself contains a chemical (we are not quite sure exactly what) that binds with an enzyme found in the intestines called CYP3A4. This enzyme is used to break down some drugs, and by binding to it the grapefruit chemical stops it working. This means that in patients on particular medications, the drugs are not breaking down and rise to very high levels in the blood. One glass of grapefruit juice is enough to suppress CYP3A4 activity by half, and the interactions can happen up to 3 days after eating or drinking grapefruit.

Certain types of oranges, such as Pomelo and Seville, can also cause similar effects, and in laboratory experiments pomegranate juice and starfruit juice have also been shown to block the CYP3AY enzyme, but whether they increase drug levels in the body isn't known.

The main drug groups affected in this way include statins (used to treat raised cholesterol levels), the blood pressure medications called calcium channel blockers, antidepressants and the drugs amiodarone, Viagra, Levitra and Cialis.

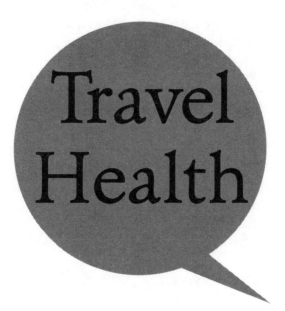

Why do I always get bitten when people in the same room aren't touched? Do mosquitoes prefer certain blood types to others?

I am the same: I get feasted on while others are totally ignored by the biting blighters. It's very unfair. A study published in *Nature* found that mosquitoes were more likely to bite people with type O blood, while people with type A got the fewest bites. Follow-up experiments examined whether this had anything to do with the fact that some people secrete chemicals related to blood type through their skin, and found that it was indeed so. Mosquitoes really favour type O 'secretors' over type O 'non-secretors' and type A secretors.

A Japanese study from 2004 let loose a swarm of hungry female mosquitoes on 64 volunteers. In true Japanese game show style, there was a twist: each mosquito had had its biting parts amputated. The researchers were able to compare how often they landed on the skin of different volunteers. They found type O secretors were twice as attractive to mosquitoes as type A secretors.

Bright sparks have come up with theories as to why this is so. Some have suggested that being infected with malaria changes your body odour or breath to attract more of the mosquitoes that infected you in the first place. But interestingly, a study by the World Health Organization showed that Indian malaria victims were more likely to have type A blood than any other type, not because people with type A get bitten more, but rather because when they do get bitten, their type A blood makes them more likely to contract malaria as a result.

Did You Know... Every 30 seconds a child dies from malaria in Africa. It is the leading cause of death in that region among under-fives.

What I can do to prevent getting bitten by mosquitoes while on holiday? Does eating Marmite really help?

Take a good insecticide spray with you when you travel and spray your room when you first arrive and then every night you're there, making sure you include under the bed, on the curtains and behind and under furniture. Use a mosquito net if one is provided.

Insects like mosquitoes bite at dawn and dusk, so use an insect repellent spray on exposed areas of skin (especially the ankles) that contains at least 50 per cent DEET, and wear long sleeves and long trousers in the evenings. This will help you avoid getting bitten. You can also buy special sprays that impregnate material to make clothes unattractive to biting insects.

Many people swear by the repellent (!) properties of Marmite, their reasoning being that it causes the skin to give off an odour which mosquitoes find unappealing. Others take high-dose B vitamin complex capsules for the same reason. Studies have not been able to back up these claims, however. The University of Connecticut did a study that proved eating garlic does not prevent one from getting bitten by mosquitoes either, and interestingly they also found that beer drinkers get even more bites than normal.

I have been on holiday to Kenya and had to take anti-malaria tablets every day. I developed really itchy patches on my skin and I burned really easily in the sun. Was that caused by my malaria medicine, and should I not take it in future?

You should always take anti-malarials if you are in a malaria zone, as it is a serious disease that can kill. In this case the risks of the disease nearly always outweigh the side-effects of the pills.

You were probably taking a drug called doxycycline, which is known to make your skin very sensitive to sunlight. It can give you itchy patches and lumps on your skin after you have been in

178

the sun, and also give your skin a bluish discolouration. In women it can cause an increase in thrush outbreaks, too. It should go away after you stop taking the drug – but remember that you must keep taking it for a month *after* you have left the malaria area. In the meantime stay out of the sun and use a high-factor sunscreen as well. If required for a future holiday, there are other anti-malaria tablets that you can take instead which don't have the same side-effects.

Is it dangerous to try for a baby or become pregnant while taking malaria tablets?

The simple answer to your question is yes, it can be dangerous to take certain anti-malaria tablets while trying for a baby because several of them have a potential to cause foetal abnormalities.

I would advise you to avoid all malaria areas if you are pregnant. Although some tablets can be taken in pregnancy, it would be better to take no unnecessary medication whatsoever, especially in the early stages of pregnancy. Malaria can be more serious in pregnant women, and the first third of pregnancy is when your baby is most at risk of the effects of anti-malaria medication.

The most commonly used medications include chloroquine and proguanil or maloprim or mefloquine. Sometimes doxycycline is used as an alternative, but all of them advise against their use in pregnancy, and even those that are less risky say only to take them if absolutely necessary.

While it is not always possible to avoid travelling to malaria areas, it is usually possible to take precautions. It would be foolish to deliberately try to conceive while taking malaria tablets, but not taking malaria tablets when living permanently in an area where the disease is endemic is equally foolish.

Top 10 Addictions of Modern Lifestyles

1) Workaholism

Very much encouraged in the modern commercial world, where every minute spent working can mean increased earnings. But all work and no play can lead to total burnout, and workaholics usually don't realize there's a problem until things go badly wrong.

2) Love Addiction

Not the same as sex addiction; the love addict can never let an infatuation go, meaning it can affect his health and relationships. Research suggests feelings of love are caused by a rise in phenylethylamine, a neurological chemical that can be addictive. It has also been found that people who are infatuated share similar symptoms with cocaine abusers, like sleeplessness and loss of a sense of time.

3) Television Addiction

We watch an average of four hours of TV a day. This means that by the age of 65 we may well have spent around nine years glued to the box. TV addicts share many clinical abuse symptoms like helplessness in putting an end to the addiction, using their 'drug of choice' to soothe their nerves, and irritability when forced to discontinue the habit.

4) Teeth-whitening Addiction

Colloquially known as 'bleaching junkies', these addicts have made teeth whitening the top requested cosmetic dental procedure, increasing by 300 per cent over the last few years. It may seem harmless but actually the consequences can be as horrible as in other addictions. Excessive teeth sensitivity, bleeding gums and transparent teeth are common complaints seen by dentists.

5) Exercise Addiction

Possibly something I should recognize in myself. Exercise addiction statistics are hard to find because it usually co-exists with eating disorders like anorexia nervosa. Like other addicts, the treadmill abusers may well sacrifice their health and social life for their addiction. A study published by *Behavioural Neuroscience* in August 2009 found similarities between excessive running and drug-abuse behaviour.

6) Oniomania

Otherwise known as shopping addiction, it's not just celebrities who are afflicted. There are oniomaniacs or compulsive shoppers in almost every neighbourhood and family. Studies suggest that compulsive buying affects more than 1 in 20 adults. This impulse to buy beyond one's needs or means has been linked to depression and has brought many shopaholics to the brink of bankruptcy.

7) Tanorexia

A silly word that has been caught up by the press, it refers to tanning addiction. We medics are concerned about tanning, and advise against the use of tanning beds, as they have been shown to be definitely carcinogenic to humans, but tanorexia continues to be a problem, especially among young women.

A 2006 study found that the UV rays of tanning beds produce feel-good endorphins in the body, falling levels of which post-tanning can trigger withdrawal symptoms similar to those caused by alcohol and drug withdrawal.

8) Sex Addiction

The craving for sexual gratification is as old as human history. But modern dysfunctional families are often blamed for turning a human urge into sexually compulsive behaviour, and some feel that easy access to Internet porn has only reinforced it. Not all psychiatrists recognize this addiction, but growing numbers of self-help groups and sex recovery centres have been set up to help treat what they see as a very real problem.

9) Internet Addiction
Constant, unstoppable, obsessive Internet browsing that becomes a daily routine, and where any interruption causes irritability, may well indicate the presence of an Internet Addiction Disorder. Psychiatrists are now acknowledging the mood-altering effects of online pornography, gambling, gaming, networking and blogging, and in some countries Internet addiction has become such a serious social problem that recovery programmes have been put in place.

10) Plastic Surgery Addiction
Negative body image is driving hordes of people under the surgeon's knife. In 2006, the British Association of Aesthetic Plastic Surgeons warned its members about patients with a body dysmorphic disorder or 'imagined ugly syndrome' for whom cosmetic surgery is an unending journey due to these addicts' dissatisfaction with the results. The organization reported an alarming study that found 40 per cent of Botox users admitting to being lured to it by the attraction of continued treatment.

Recently while on holiday in Cambodia I was scratched by the sharp tooth of a puppy. It didn't bleed at all but has left a small mark. I was vaccinated for rabies but am wondering if I now need to go and get treatment for exposure to rabies?

I don't think this will be necessary, first because you have already had a course of rabies jabs, and secondly because no blood was drawn and you have no symptoms. If you had never had any rabies vaccines, then I would be suggesting that you talk to a specialist about your risk after this puppy incident.

This really highlights the importance of making sure all of your vaccines are up to date before you travel, as well as having any jabs pertinent to your final destination.

Did You Know... In China, 300 million smokers devour approximately 1.7 trillion cigarettes a year, or 3 million cigarettes a minute. This explains the fact that 1.2 million people in China die from smoking each year – that's 2,000 people a day.

Can frequent flying cause cancer?

The World Health Organization is worried about the risk of cancer among regular flyers following research that showed that flight attendants were twice as likely to get skin cancer and 30 per cent more likely to get breast cancer than the general population. These figures could possibly be the result of lifestyle rather than airline travel, but with the average long-haul flight attendant being exposed to radiation equal to 250 chest X-rays each year, one can see that there is a cause for concern. But very few travellers fly as often as cabin crew, so this risk is much reduced for the majority. My advice is to take proactive measures such as not overexposing your skin to the sun and, for women, making sure you regularly check your breasts for changes and go see your doctor if you find any.

Did You Know... Scientists have developed more than 150 antibiotics to help stop the spread of infectious diseases.

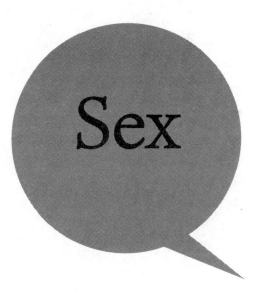

My mother told me that masturbating will make me go blind, but I still do it. How long have I got until my eyes go?

I can't really believe that I need to answer this one! If I told you that 95 per cent of men and women masturbate, and the other 5 per cent are lying, would you feel better? If your mother were right there would be very few sighted people on this planet. It doesn't give you hairy palms, either...

Many societies have decided that masturbation is a shameful, embarrassing, 'dirty' behaviour that should be discouraged. This couldn't be further from the truth. Doctors think masturbation is healthy as it relieves stress and feels good. Masturbation may also help to prevent prostate cancer. A study done in Australia in 2003 showed that men who masturbated regularly in their twenties were a third less likely to develop aggressive prostate cancer later in life. The theory is that frequent ejaculation prevents carcinogens from building up in the prostate and causing cancers to form over a period of time. So while I suspect that an obsession with masturbation could result in some unpleasant side-effects, including chafing, in general nothing bad will happen if you do it.

I have got a new girlfriend, but when we have sex I can't keep my erection. Why?

If this is this the first time you've experienced this and you can get erections at other times, then this is probably situational and psychological. The more you worry about it, the more it will happen. Sex therapists would recommend that you and your girlfriend agree a limit: meaning you can do anything you like with each other sexually except penetration. Do this for the next few weeks and you may find that erections can then comfortably be developed and maintained because you don't reach the 'pressure' point. As you then become comfortable with each other sexually, things should go well when you drop the self-imposed limit. It's a simple but often effective method, but if it doesn't work then go and see your GP or a family planning clinic. The sooner it's dealt with, the better.

What should I do if I think I'm gay?

Um, nothing! Your sexual identity usually develops over time, and figuring out your sexuality can be a tricky process. For some people, being gay is something they work out from an early age. For others, it can take much longer, and you may not fully realize and understand your feelings until later in life. Many people have feelings towards other people of the same sex, though having these thoughts and feelings does not necessarily mean that they are gay. Taking your time to figure out your sexuality is perfectly normal and whatever you decide you are is fine – celebrate it.

Did You Know... On any given day, sexual intercourse takes place 120 million times on earth. About 4 per cent of the world's population are having sex on any given day.

Sex can be very painful and my vagina gets sore and tender straight after. This has been going on for a while now. What could it be?

Pain during sex, called *dyspareunia*, can cause a vicious cycle to occur in which you start to fear sex and so become tense, tightening your vaginal muscles and making any pain worse. Common causes include anxiety, lack of relaxation or lubrication, dry vagina due to hormonal changes, infections like thrush or bacterial vaginosis (BV) and injuries such as tearing during childbirth. Pain on deep penetration may be caused by inflammation of the pelvic organs caused by endometriosis, cysts, pelvic inflammatory disease or even irritable bowel syndrome. The best thing is to see your GP for a full check-up; he or she may decide to refer you to a gynaecologist if the cause is not immediately obvious.

I am 48 and have a really low sex drive. I'm just not interested in it any more. Why is this happening?

You should try to work out if it is just sex that seems to hold no interest for you or if it's most things in life in general, which could indicate that you are depressed. Checks of your hormone levels including your thyroid and testosterone levels may be useful, and looking at any drugs or medications that you are taking may offer a clue. Lifestyle, stress and lack of sleep will all contribute. Talk to your GP to help you work out the cause.

I find it impossible to maintain an erection if I am wearing a condom. I have tried different sizes but this makes little difference. Is there any possible explanation for this?

This is quite a common problem for a lot of men, so much so that we doctors encounter men with this problem several times a week. It is most often due to anxiety. At the very moment the man starts to roll the condom onto his penis, his brain starts to worry about whether he'll be stiff enough to 'fill' the condom. The body instantly starts producing anxiety chemicals and these stop the erection.

One solution is to get your partner to put the condom on you, stimulating you by hand at the same time. If this doesn't work after several attempts, then seek counselling to try to diminish your anxiety in sexual situations.

I can't bear to let anything penetrate me and have been unable to have relationships because of this. I can't even use tampons for the same reasons. Will I ever be able to have sex?

It is very likely you have a condition called vaginismus, which causes the muscles of the vagina to tense and spasm, preventing any sort of penetration. You should still be able to get aroused and even orgasm through stimulation of your clitoris, however. To overcome this, a psychosexual counsellor may help. Treatment can involve gradual desensitizing techniques to help you get comfortable with objects on and eventually in your vagina. The cure rate with a good counsellor is very high, so there is every chance you will get this sorted.

Did You Know... The largest cell in the human body is the female egg, and the smallest is the male sperm. The ovum is typically large enough to be seen with the naked eye, with a diameter of about 1 millimetre. The sperm cell, on the other hand, is tiny, consisting of little more than nucleus.

I've been in a relationship for eight years and, after recurring bouts of cystitis, have just tested positive for chlamydia. Does this mean my partner must have cheated on me?

Chlamydia is a very common sexually transmitted infection: around 1 in 10 women is thought to carry it, but it is usually symptom-free, which means you can have it for years without knowing. So the fact you have it doesn't necessarily mean your partner has been sleeping around. Nevertheless, you do need to sit down and talk about it, as it's important that you both get treated with antibiotics or you'll just pass it back and forth. Left untreated, it can cause pelvic inflammatory disease and damage your fertility, so you need to get it sorted.

What are warts and why do we get them?

A virus called the human papilloma virus (HPV) causes the warts that you can get on your hands as well as anal and genital warts. There are about 100 different types of this virus and they cause the different kinds of warts that occur on different parts of the body. The virus is mainly spread by skin-to-skin contact. Although this is often during sex in the case of genital warts, it doesn't absolutely have to be. We know that the virus can survive outside the body, and so in theory it may be possible to catch warts without close contact, but in practice there have not been any proven recorded cases of this happening and so I would say that it is pretty unlikely that you would catch, say, genital warts in a sauna without physical contact with other people. An example of a wart that can be transmitted without direct contact is the verruca – these are warts that infect the skin on your feet and are often caught in swimming pools or gyms.

Warts are not just unsightly. The virus can also cause various different cancers including penile and anal cancers, and cervical cancer in women. Ask your sexual health clinic for more information and to check you if you are concerned, and always use condoms for sex. Having said this, condoms are not totally protective against the wart virus.

Two HPV vaccines have been developed that protect against some of the more serious cancer-causing virus types. They are mainly aimed at girls to try to protect them from cervical cancer, but if given to boys may help to reduce the risk of anal cancers, too.

What tests and treatments are available for erectile problems?

There can be many causes of erectile problems and so tests need to be quite broad based to find the problem. They include a good chat with your doctor which may identify the problem by itself, a genital examination, urine and blood tests, and sometimes a blood supply test where the flow of blood to the penis is assessed, usually by inducing an erection using a drug.

The best treatment depends on the cause. Many cases of erectile dysfunction are due to psychological issues, but physical treatments include medications like sildenafil (Viagra) and apomorphine (Uprima), injections into the penis (Viridal and Caverject), urethral pellets such as MUSE (medical urethral system of erection), hormonal treatment (testosterone replacement therapy), vacuum devices (battery-operated suction pump), counselling and cognitive therapy (couples or relationship therapy), psychosexual therapy using the sensate focus technique, and surgery (penile implant).

Did You Know... The three things pregnant women dream most of during their first trimester are frogs, worms and potted plants. Pregnancy hormones can cause mood swings, cravings and many other unexpected changes.

What can I do to avoid getting problems with erections?

Most men experience erection problems at one time or another. It's a very common issue most often due to stress, alcohol or tiredness, and improves with time. It is more common in men aged 40–70, and in the majority of cases an underlying physical cause can be found, although emotional and psychological factors may also be involved, too. Fewer than 20 per cent of cases are purely psychological.

The most common causes are ageing combined with arteriosclerosis (hardening of the arteries) and smoking, but also diabetes, drug misuse, Alzheimer's disease, Parkinson's disease, hormone deficiency, kidney failure, Peyronie's disease, neurological disorders such as multiple sclerosis, spinal or back injuries, and other long-term illnesses. Psychological conditions such as depression, anxiety, stress and trauma may contribute. Relationship issues can play a part: performance anxiety, poor communication, sexual inexperience, reduced attraction, fear of intimacy and infidelity. Medication, alcohol, smoking and the use of antidepressants and antihypertensives are culprits and, rarely, hormonal conditions like having abnormally low levels of the male hormone testosterone, or producing too much of the pituitary hormone prolactin.

To decrease your chances of this becoming a regular problem for you, it's important not to smoke or drink excessively. Try to exercise regularly and eat well, making sure you get plenty of fruit and veg. Try to keep your stress levels low – if you do experience stress or depression, speak to your GP for advice, and try to get plenty of sleep. Have regular medical screenings and check-ups to make sure problems like diabetes, high blood pressure and high cholesterol are detected early so treatments can be offered.

What do I do if my erection won't go down?

The medical name for an erection that won't go down is a *priapism*. It can be a nuisance, as it is more likely to occur when you don't have any sexual desire than when you want a long-lasting erection. It can also damage the tissues in the penis, and is usually extremely painful. It occurs because the blood in the penis, which gives you the erection, cannot escape. This happens because of prolonged sexual desire or as a side-effect of some types of medication. Sometimes it can be because medication for impotence has worked too well. Rarely, it is because of an underlying condition such as sickle-cell anaemia or a prostate problem. If your erection lasts for three to four hours or more, it is likely to be priapism and you should get urgent medical attention. If it has lasted less than four a doctor can usually treat it with decongestant medicines, but if you have had an erection for longer than six hours, a doctor will usually need to release blood from the penis using a needle and syringe. The doctor will also try to find out the cause of your priapism and treat you for this, if necessary. In some cases, surgery may be required to avoid causing permanent damage to the penis.

When I come it can give me a cramping pain near my bottom, I've had it for a month or so now. What is causing it?

This can be a typical symptom of prostatitis – an inflammation of the prostate gland. Other symptoms include a strong feeling of the need to pee and generalized pains around the penis and bottom. A bacterial infection, sometimes starting in the bladder and then ending up in the prostate, often causes it, and can be treated with antibiotics. If you have had a new sexual partner or partners, then get a sexual health screen and advice from your doctor. Sometimes you may need to take antibiotics for several months before it clears completely.

10 Facts You May Not Know About the Orgasm

1)   Somebody who clearly had too much time on their hands calculated that the average male will orgasm enough fluid over his lifetime to fill 94 pint glasses!

2)   It's not just women who have various g-spot locations. Men have them, too – three to be precise, but relatively few men discover them all. They are the frenulum (small fold of tissue under the glans penis), the perineum (the area between the testicles and anus), and the prostate gland.

3)   For most guys an orgasm is good at any time, but for women there seem to be certain times that are better than others. Rather unfortunately, her best orgasms are often experienced during her period, but this is not well known as most couples avoid sex during this time. The reason for the enhanced orgasm is thought to be due to the increase in blood circulation around the groin area at this time.

4)   Marilyn Monroe never had one. But she gave a famous description of her sexual experiences to her psychiatrist: 'Think of a light switch with a rheostat control. As you begin to turn it on, the bulb begins to get bright, then brighter, and brighter and finally in a blinding flash is fully lit. It is so good.' Sounds like she may have got close, at least.

5)   The average speed of the ejaculate shooting out during a male orgasm is 28 mph. In contrast, the sperm it contains are only capable of travelling approximately 10cm per hour. The force of the orgasm is thought to give them a head start, considering they have several centimetres to go before they reach their final destination.

6) OK, this one is rather morbid, but it's not just the living who have orgasms. If you electronically stimulate and oxygenate the sacral nerves in the spinal cord of a dead body you can cause it to climax. I don't want to even begin to think about how and why that was ever discovered.

7) The amount of noise a woman makes during sex has a significant effect on the success of the male orgasm. It's the more overtly vocal women who achieve the desired results on a consistent basis. Studies show that men orgasm 59 per cent of the time while their partner is screaming in ecstasy, and only 2 per cent of the time if she lies there quietly. I suspect it has a lot to do with stimulating the male ego ...

8) Some think that women have a much harder time than men when it comes to basic biological functions. But one reward is their ability to have multiple orgasms. The most female orgasms recorded were 134 in a single hour. There are some medical conditions that can cause women to experience multiple orgasms without sexual contact, merely by stroking their eyebrow, rubbing their knee, thinking about sex or even brushing their teeth.

9) The anthropologist Desmond Morris famously theorized on the evolutionary reason for the female orgasm. He suggested its purpose was not only to encourage interest in sex, but also to promote exhaustion, encouraging her to remain lying down to prevent sperm from leaking out. He also suggested that some women's difficulty in attaining orgasm with certain men was also built in on purpose: only the most patient, caring and imaginative men would have the best chance of eliciting an orgasm, and thus successfully conceiving a child, and this sort of man must surely make a better father. Not all agree.

10) While the Catholic Church will undoubtedly refute it, masturbatory actions have been seen in prenatal ultrasound images, especially in males. The hand can be seen wrapped around the penis and moving respectively back and forth. It is not uncommon to find young children engaging in various forms of self-stimulation, resulting in a sort of orgasm.

I find sex quite uncomfortable and my GP said it is because I have a retroverted uterus. I obviously can't do much about that, but can I make sex any better?

Having a retroverted uterus means it tips backwards rather than forwards, the more common position, but it may not necessarily be this that is causing your discomfort. Many women experience some pain and pressure on deep penetration, probably due to the sensitivity of the internal organs. You can improve your sex life simply by trying different sexual positions. Try being on top so that you can control the depth of penetration, or when you are on your back, keep your legs down flat. A bit of experimentation with an eager partner (not too hard to find) should help you find a position that suits.

Did You Know... Your teeth start growing six months before you are born. At nine to twelve weeks, the foetus starts to form the teeth buds that will turn into baby teeth.

I hear that sportspeople like footballers and top athletes are told not to have sex the night before a big game as it can affect their performance. Is there any truth in this?

This is advice that is often circulated, and that everyone has heard of, but there is no truth in it whatsoever. The theory behind it is that not having sex will increase testosterone and aggression levels, and so will improve sporting performance, but research does not support this. In fact, many athletes I know say it makes no difference whether they have sex or not, and certainly don't avoid it on purpose before big events. As sex is one of nature's most effective sleeping pills, it would seem that it might help with any nerves and anxiety the night before, and so ensure a good night's sleep.

Is gonorrhoea only ever sexually transmitted? My daughter got it and I was horrified that she was even having sex. Is there no other way it could have occurred?

The answer to this really depends on what your definition of 'sexually transmitted' is. In the vast majority of cases gonorrhoea is transmitted from one person to another by sexual contact, be it vaginal, anal or oral sex – but not in every case. I know of several doctors working in sexual health clinics who gave themselves gonorrhoea after touching infected patients – in a non-sexual way, of course. It is also known to have been transmitted via shared use of an inflatable sex doll with an artificial vagina that was not washed between use. On the other hand, and despite much research into whether it's possible to catch STIs from toilet seats, repeated testing has failed to isolate the gonorrhoea bacteria (gonococcus). There was, however, a case reported of an 8-year-old girl who contracted it, most probably through using a very dirty toilet on an overcrowded plane in Russia. It was probably picked up on her fingers, which she then touched herself with while wiping after using the toilet. While the bacteria cannot survive well in a dry environment outside the body, it has been known to survive for short periods on plastic, and so could, in theory, be transmitted on shared sex toys.

My new girlfriend says she gets something called BV and cystitis from time to time. Is it dangerous for me?

The vagina normally has a balance of 'good' bacteria and (fewer) 'harmful' bacteria. Bacterial vaginosis, or BV, develops when this balance changes, causing an increase in harmful bacteria and a decrease in good bacteria. It is unlikely that you will catch this from your girlfriend as BV does not usually affect men in any way, and is not sexually transmitted.

As for cystitis, this is otherwise known as a urinary tract infection and could well be caused by a bacteria found on our own bodies, rather than from any sexual transmission. The sensible thing to do is to use a condom, or avoid sex until this infection is cured.

Did You Know... Babies are, pound for pound, stronger than oxen. While a baby certainly couldn't pull a covered wagon at its present size, if the child were the size of an ox it just might very well be able to. Babies have especially strong and powerful legs for such tiny creatures.

Is sperm actually alive?

Yes. A single sperm is really an independent single-celled organism, a bit like an amoeba. In fact it is more alive than any other cell in the male body, as it's the only one that can reproduce.

I come very quickly during sex. It is very frustrating and affects my relationships. Why does it happen?

Premature ejaculation is certainly one of the most common sexual problems. Approximately 10 per cent of males have experienced it at some time. It's more common in younger men as it tends to improve with age. There is no set definition, but as a rule the average 'lasting time' of men with premature ejaculation is 1.8 minutes, whereas the average time for men not affected by PE is 7.3 minutes.

One of the more popular theories about why it happens has to do with early conditioning. Rushed and furtive early sexual experiences condition the sufferer to climax as quickly as possible, and this then carries on into his later experiences.

While I am aware that this next bit of info is not really going to make you feel any better, it's worth knowing that, from an evolutionary point of view, males who ejaculated quickly were more likely to have children, as they stood more chance of impregnating a woman.

There may also be an inherited aspect to this, as it can run in families, which is a counter-argument to the conditioning theory.

Anxiety or 'nerves' definitely play a part in many cases as well. If you're nervous, you're likely to come too quickly.

What can I do to stop me coming too quickly?

You have a lot of options. If you have very mild premature ejaculation (PE), then simple distraction techniques may help. This means turning your mind to something else when you sense that climax is near. For example, you can think about something totally unconcerned with sex, or pinch yourself.

Local anaesthetic gels are available to desensitize the penis and dampen down sexual sensation. They can work, but the problem is that the gels also desensitize the partner, too – not often desired. You can get condoms that contain a local anaesthetic (benzocaine) inside them that will have the same effect, or more simply you could try wearing extra safe (and therefore extra thick) condoms to achieve the same effect.

The American therapists Masters and Johnson developed a special 'penis grip' technique that involves both partners. It involves your partner squeezing the glans of your penis firmly when you feel you are near orgasm. This abolishes the desire to climax, so if you use it over a period of weeks, you can usually re-train yourself to last much longer.

A newer treatment involves taking an antidepressant drug a few hours before intercourse. Delaying male climax is a well-known side-effect of certain antidepressants and, while not usually an upside, for guys with premature ejaculation it's a positive boon. Antidepressants that are commonly used for this purpose include clomipramine, fluoxetine and sertraline; ask your GP if you feel they may help you.

There is yet another possibility you could try: the stop-start technique. When masturbating, stop when you are near the point of ejaculation. Let the feeling subside and then continue to masturbate. Do this three times, and finally allow yourself to ejaculate on the fourth time. Because there are often psychological difficulties as well as behavioural and mechanical ones, you will probably benefit more from seeking treatment rather than using the stop-start technique on its own.

Did You Know… Every human spent about half an hour as a single cell. All life has to begin somewhere, and even the largest humans spent a short part of their lives as a single-celled organism when sperm and egg cells first combined.

I recently kissed a guy, and noticed he had a small amount of blood on the front of his front teeth. I'm now really worried that I could catch HIV from this. What should I do?

It would be *very* unusual and unlikely for HIV to be transmitted to you by what you did. While in theory it is possible that blood from someone with HIV could be infectious in this way, the reality is that HIV is simply not transmitted through kissing. Also remember that the blood you saw could actually have come from you.

Even oral sex is considered low risk for catching HIV. Stomach acid deactivates the virus and so, provided you are not exposed to a lot of semen, you are not at high risk. It is so unlikely that you could absorb enough of someone's blood via kissing to infect you under most normal circumstances that you do not need to worry. Avoiding HIV is really very simple: use condoms.

Which body fluids can transmit the HIV virus, and which ones can't?

This is very straightforward: blood, pre-cum, semen, vaginal secretions and breast milk all contain high concentrations of HIV, and all have been linked to transmission of the virus.

Saliva, tears, sweat and urine can have the virus in them, but in such small concentrations that nobody has ever been infected through them. However, if any body fluid is visibly contaminated with blood, the risk of transmission exists.

Can I get HIV from oral sex?

Yes, it is possible to become infected with HIV through performing or receiving oral sex, but the risk is low. There have been a few documented cases. While no one knows exactly what the degree of risk is, evidence suggests that it is certainly much less than that of unprotected anal or vaginal sex.

If you are receiving oral sex from someone else, you are only being exposed to saliva. The concentrations of the virus in saliva are so low that nobody has ever been infected from saliva. If giving someone oral sex there is a risk of becoming infected, since pre-cum, semen, vaginal secretions and menstrual blood can get into the mouth. The more of these body fluids you are exposed to, the greater the risk of infection. Of course, the virus must also be able to get into your bloodstream through some type of open sore, abrasion, gum disease, etc. So the more cuts or open sores in your mouth, or the more gum disease you have, the greater the risk would be.

As a general rule, no exposure to pre-cum or semen equals no risk as far as HIV is concerned. Exposure to pre-cum only equals a low risk (but is still technically possible). The more pre-cum you get exposed to, the greater the risk would be. Exposure to both pre-cum and semen is risky, especially if there are cuts/open sores in the mouth.

The risk of HIV transmission also increases if the person giving or receiving oral sex has another sexually transmitted disease.

Contraception, Fertility & Hormones

If I am breastfeeding I can't get pregnant, right?

In theory this is true, but in practice it doesn't always work out that way. The theory is that breastfeeding releases prolactin, a hormone that can suppress certain stages of the menstrual cycle. As long as prolactin levels are high, for example while you are exclusively breastfeeding a new baby, then your normal menstrual cycle won't occur. It's true that women who exclusively breastfeed their babies do not have any periods until they stop breastfeeding altogether or introduce some bottle-feeds on a regular basis, but not all women breastfeed exclusively and regularly enough to keep the cycle suppressed. Any woman with a regular menstrual cycle can become pregnant, and since many women get their first postpartum period while they're still lactating, they could get pregnant again during this time. So generally it's not a good idea to rely on breastfeeding as your only form of contraception. If you have started having sex again then it's important to use an additional form of contraception.

How effective is contraception?

Some methods of contraception are more effective at preventing pregnancy than others, but this is provided you follow the instructions and use them correctly. This is often where many people fall down. No contraceptive is 100 per cent reliable, and some can have side-effects.

Condoms are about 98 per cent effective if used correctly. Diaphragms and caps with spermicide are 92–96 per cent effective if used correctly.

The combined contraceptive pill is over 99 per cent effective if taken correctly, as is the progestogen-only pill. Contraceptive injections are also over 99 per cent effective. They last for 8 or 12 weeks, depending on the type of injection.

Intrauterine systems (containing some locally-released hormone) and intrauterine devices (IUDs) are over 99 per cent effective. They can stay in place for 5–10 years, depending on the type, but can also be taken out at any time.

Withdrawal before ejaculation and natural family planning are notoriously unreliable, especially for women whose periods are very irregular.

Did You Know... Recent American research suggests that almost one-third of men of all ages say they climax too early, and nearly one-fifth of men in their fifties experience problems achieving or maintaining an erection.

When can I use contraception again after having a baby?

It's possible to become pregnant again very soon after the birth of a baby, even if you're breastfeeding and even if your periods haven't returned. You ovulate about two weeks before your period arrives, so your fertility may return sooner than you think.

You can use condoms as soon as you feel ready to have sex again, but I wouldn't rush into things. The combined pill, progestogen-only pill and contraceptive implants can all be used from 21 days after the birth, but the combined pill is not recommended if you are breastfeeding, as it can affect your milk supply. An IUD or IUS can usually be fitted six to eight weeks after giving birth.

What should I do if I miss a pill?

This is rather a complex question. It depends on what type of contraceptive pill you are taking, and how many pills you have missed. If you are unsure about what to do if you have missed a pill, ring your local Family Planning Clinic or visit an NHS Walk-in

Centre for individual advice. In the UK you can also call Sexual Health Direct on 0845 122 8690, or consult any GP or pharmacist. If you are still having sex then I would certainly use extra protection like condoms until you have been given advice.

When will my periods return after stopping the Pill?

It can take a while for your periods to come back after you stop taking the Pill. For most women it's two to four weeks before you have a period, but this varies from woman to woman and also depends on what your cycle is normally like. Weight, health, stress, how much exercise you take and whether you have conditions such as polycystic ovarian syndrome (PCOS) can all influence the cycle of periods.

Your periods may be irregular when you first come off the Pill, and you should allow up to 6 months for your natural cycle to re-establish itself fully. It's quite common to have a longer delay before normal periods start again after stopping the Pill, especially if you have run two or three packets together. This is because the Pill contains the hormones that stop ovulation (the release of an egg) each month.

How will I know if I have reached the menopause if I am taking the Pill?

The menopause is the time when your periods permanently cease. The average age for the menopause is 50–51, with the perimenopause (the years preceding the menopause) starting around the age of 46–47. Contraception is necessary until the menopause. It is advised that contraception should continue to be used until you have not had a period or any bleeding for two years if you are aged under 50, and for one year if you are over 50.

Taking the combined contraceptive pill may mask the menopause by controlling menopausal symptoms such as hot flushes and night sweats. Therefore, it may be difficult to assess when you are no longer fertile. There is no test that can absolutely establish when the menopause has occurred, but your doctor can measure the level of the hormone oestrogen (which will be low) and of the hormone FSH (which will be raised) in perimenopausal and menopausal women. This blood test should be planned for the last day of the Pill-free interval.

Top 10 Amazing Facts about Breasts

1)   The world's biggest fake boobs are a size 38KKK. They took nine surgeries and more than a gallon of silicone.

2)   GoTopless.org is an organization claiming that women should have the same constitutional right to go bare-chested in public as men. They often promote topless gatherings to claim for their rights, which unsurprisingly attract a large (mostly male) audience.

3)   No two breasts are exactly the same size and the left breast is usually bigger than the right one. Nipples also come in varying sizes and can point in different directions, too.

4)   Research has shown that breasts are often the first things that men look at, and for a longer time than any other body part. I'm not so sure that research needed to be commissioned to work that one out. Interestingly, another study found that staring at women's breasts for a few minutes each day can improve a man's health and can add four or five years to his life!

5)   Men can lactate, too. They have mammary glands, which under the influence of certain hormones can produce milk.

6)   A survey by a bra manufacturer found that British women have the largest breasts in Europe. More than half the women in the UK wear a D cup. Italian women were found to have the smallest breasts.

7)   The average breast weighs about 1kg and makes up about 4–5 per cent of body fat.

8) Young breasts are made up of fat, milk glands and collagen, but as they age the glands and collagen shrink, being replaced by more and more fat. This is why breasts droop downwards with age.

9) Women who get breast implants are at least three times more likely to commit suicide. This is because it has been found that women who undergo breast surgery have a higher incidence of psychiatric problems.

10) In Hong Kong you can get a degree in Bra Studies, which teaches you how to design and build a bra.

What is the male pill?

The male pill is a proposed new form of hormonal contraception for men. It aims to allow men to control their fertility in a similar way that the female contraceptive pill does for women, except that it probably won't actually be a pill. It will more likely be a regular injection. It uses synthetic hormones to temporarily stop sperm developing.

Scientists have been researching male contraception for some years, but more research is needed to assess its long-term safety and effectiveness. The current choice of contraception for men is limited to using condoms or having a vasectomy.

Did You Know... Every day an adult body produces 300 billion new cells, constantly repairing and building new cells to maintain your body.

Can I get my vasectomy reversed on the NHS?

A vasectomy or 'male sterilization' involves cutting the tubes that carry sperm from the testes to the penis. This prevents sperm getting from the testes to the semen that is ejaculated during orgasm.

A vasectomy is usually considered to be a permanent form of contraception because it is not always possible to reverse the procedure, which would involve re-joining the sperm-carrying tubes that were cut, or blocked, during your vasectomy. They are not usually available on the NHS. It is possible to have a vasectomy reversal carried out privately, but it may cost several thousand pounds. The problem with the procedure is that success rates are not very high, and there is no guarantee that your fertility will return.

I've been taking the Pill for around 10 years now. I've always stopped for a month each year. But will taking the Pill for such a long time interfere with my chances of getting pregnant in the future?

Every woman reacts differently to changing or stopping the Pill but, however long you have been taking it, it should have no long-term effect on your fertility at all.

After stopping the Pill it may take several months before your body returns to a normal regular cycle, and there is also a very 'rough and ready' guide that says that for every year you have been taking the Pill continuously, it will take that many months after stopping it before conceiving. This is not based on firm evidence but is often quoted by women and serves as a good rough guide. Your periods may gradually increase in flow again, too, over this time.

I had unprotected sex on the second day of my period. I have heard that you are least likely to become pregnant when you are having a period. Is this true or do I need to be worried now?

It is pretty unlikely that you would get pregnant on the second day of your period, but it is not absolutely impossible. The average menstrual cycle is 28 days, counting day 1 as the first day of menstrual bleeding. Your period comes if an egg fails to get fertilized, usually about 12 to 14 days after the egg is produced. Therefore, in the average 28-day cycle, the egg is produced around day 14. The least likely time to conceive is from day 1 to day 7, but things can always go slightly differently to how we expect them to. If in doubt I would go and talk to your doctor about whether you should take the morning-after pill if you do not want to get pregnant.

Can you tell me when I would be at my most fertile? Which stage of my cycle?

The length of a woman's menstrual cycle can vary from between 24 to 35 days, but on average it lasts 28 days. Ovulation, when an egg is released from your ovaries into your fallopian tube, occurs approximately halfway through your menstrual cycle – roughly 14 days before the start of your next period. The days around ovulation (between 10 and 16 days before your next period) are when you are at your most fertile. So if you are trying to get pregnant, this is the best time of the month to have unprotected sex with your partner.

After ejaculation, sperm can live for at least 48 hours and up to seven days inside your vagina or womb. This means that it is possible for you to become pregnant if you have had unprotected sex two days before, or a couple of days after, ovulation – that is, between days 10 and 16 of your menstrual cycle. The least likely time that you will conceive is between days 1 and 7 of your menstrual cycle.

You can buy special ovulation prediction kits, which test your temperature or hormone levels to find out when you are at your most fertile.

Did You Know... Most men have erections every hour to hour and a half during sleep. Most people's bodies and minds are much more active when they're sleeping than they think. The combination of blood circulation and testosterone production can cause erections during sleep, and they're often a normal and necessary part of REM sleep.

How can I improve my chances of getting my wife pregnant?

Your testicles produce the best sperm when they're cool. Ideally, sperm should be around 34.5°C/94.1°F, which is just below body temperature. It has been reported that wearing loose-fitting boxer shorts rather than tight-fitting Y-fronts or shorts could actually help to keep your testicles and sperm cooler and therefore of the best possible quality. Swapping steaming hot baths for a lukewarm bath or shower will also help. Smoking can reduce fertility, so make the decision to quit the fags today if you want to make a baby. Heavy drinking is known to have a negative effect on sperm quality, and this makes a successful pregnancy much less likely, so try to keep your drinking down. The recommended limit is three or four units per day for a man, so make that your maximum, and try to make it less if you can. Remember, one unit is the equivalent of half a pint of lager, a small glass of wine or one pub measure of spirits.

The best advice is for you and your partner to have lots of sex. Regular sex, especially around the time that your partner ovulates, is the best way to improve your chances of conception.

Is early menopause hereditary? My mother went through the menopause when she was about 37, and I'm concerned this will happen to me – I am 23.

Is there any way of prolonging fertility if early menopause is likely?

A tendency to early menopause does seem to run in some families. The fact that your mother went through an early menopause at 37 makes you slightly more likely to have an early menopause than someone whose mother had a later one.

In most women, the menopause occurs between 45 and 55 years, and in spite of your mother's early menopause it is still more likely that your menopause will occur within these limits.

Unfortunately there is no way of predicting when your menopause will occur, and there is no way of prolonging your fertility if you are destined to have an early menopause.

Can the contraceptive pill affect your libido? Since starting taking one I have had no sex drive whatsoever.

The majority of different contraceptive pills available have oestrogen in them as standard, but contain different progestogens. It is these progestogens that can cause libido problems like the ones you are experiencing.

Lack of libido is often caused not by one problem alone, however, and may be part and parcel of relationship issues. Perhaps you should reflect on your relationship a little and ask yourself if there are any problems there that might be affecting your desire.

If all seems well then you could try changing pills to one with a different progestogen and seeing if after a few months things have improved.

You read a lot about the risks of HRT in older women, but what are the risks for younger women on HRT like me? Am I at risk of osteoporosis or breast cancer?

I think I should point out straight away that there is no such thing as a risk-free or side-effect-free drug. One has to make a decision based on the outcome of assessing whether the risks outweigh the benefits.

The main body of research has focused primarily on risks in older women – but those same risks will apply to younger women, too.

The big difference, however, is in the benefits, which are far greater in younger women who have undergone a premature menopause for whatever reason, than in older women. So doing our risk-versus-benefit calculation for you I would confidently say that the benefits of taking HRT outweigh the harms in your particular age group.

Did You Know... The number of multiple births has increased by more than 400 per cent in the last 20 years.

I have been taking HRT for a few years and want to know if it would be OK to have unprotected sex without the risk of pregnancy?

This is a very common question but the answer really depends on your own particular circumstance.

Most HRT tablets do not have any contraceptive effect. You may well be having a monthly bleed in response to the hormone cycle supplied by your pills, but this does not necessarily indicate fertility. If your periods had stopped for more than a year before you started HRT, then you have almost certainly gone through the menopause and so won't need contraception. If, however, you were still having periods when you started HRT then it is impossible to know whether you have gone through the menopause or not, or whether there might still be a chance that you could conceive.

The only way to know for sure would be to stop the HRT for a period of time and see whether your periods return. If they don't, you can be quite sure that you have gone through the menopause and you don't need to use contraception. If your periods return, this would suggest that you are still ovulating and could become pregnant.

Can hormones cause depression? If you are on the Pill or taking HRT, could that give you depression?

Depression is a common problem in women going through the menopause. Hormone replacement therapy is designed to do exactly what it says: to replace the hormones that are lost during the menopause, and therefore prevent the symptoms and adverse effects of the menopause like hot flushes, irregular menstruation, breast tenderness and loss of libido, as well as depression. The lack of female hormones after the menopause also leads to an increase in the incidence of osteoporosis, heart attacks and strokes.

There are many different types and strengths of Pill and HRT available, and sometimes it takes a considerable time and numerous changes to get just the right balance for a particular woman.

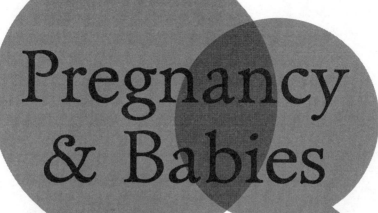

What's the best baby-making position? Am I more likely to fall pregnant in some positions than in others?

I can honestly say that countless studies have been done on this topic and all have found that position makes no difference at all. Standing on your head afterwards is not much use, either. Getting pregnant is really all about timing. You need to make sure you are having sex during your most fertile period, which is normally between days 10 and 16 for a woman with the average 28-day cycle, where day 1 is the start of your last period. I think trying different positions will help you to keep the love-making going, however, and keep it interesting, which can only help!

What is an ectopic pregnancy?

An ectopic pregnancy is one that develops outside the womb. In a normal pregnancy, an egg is released from one of the woman's ovaries. It travels down a narrow passage called a fallopian tube, which connects the ovaries to the womb. The egg is fertilized by a sperm from the man and is implanted in the lining of the womb, where it grows into a baby. In an ectopic pregnancy, the fertilized egg implants outside the womb. In most ectopic pregnancies it implants in one of the narrow fallopian tubes. Many ectopic pregnancies end in a natural miscarriage very early on, and the woman may never even know she was pregnant, but in some cases the growing embryo can split or tear the fallopian tube, causing serious internal bleeding.

Signs that your pregnancy might be ectopic include cramps and bleeding, and severe pain, on one side of your lower abdomen.

I have just had a baby and my boyfriend wants to start having sex again but I'm still sore and not in the mood. Is it safe to start having sex soon after giving birth?

I always tell my female patients not to even consider having full sex until after the postnatal check-up, which usually takes place about six weeks after the birth. If you have needed stitches and you are still sore, then you will not be ready even then. If you do start then please use plenty of extra lubrication. Don't expect things to get straight back to normal as childbirth most definitely does affect your sex life. You will be experiencing hormone changes and emotional stresses, and very few women feel sexy until a long time after they have given birth. This may take six months or so to sort itself out, so be prepared and tell him to be patient.

Did You Know... Tuesday is the most popular day for babies to make their arrival in the world.

How can I make sure my baby doesn't die of cot death? The thought terrifies me.

Cot death, also known as sudden infant death syndrome (SIDS), is the sudden and unexpected death of an infant. Some 90 per cent of cot deaths occur in infants under six months of age. Although it is not known exactly what causes cot death, there are several steps that can be taken to reduce the risks. Never smoke around your baby. This includes fathers and anyone else who may live in your home. Don't let anyone smoke in the same room as your baby, or near your baby if you are out, for example in a café or restaurant. Place your baby on his back to sleep, not on his front or side, and don't let him get too hot. Breastfeed if you can, and it is OK to settle your baby to sleep with a dummy – it does not matter if the dummy falls out while he is asleep.

For the first six months, the safest place for your baby to sleep is in a cot in your bedroom. One study found that over half (52 per cent) of the cot deaths investigated might have been prevented if the baby had slept in his parents' room, but not in their bed.

What are pelvic floor exercises? My midwife told me I need to start doing them.

The pelvic floor muscles are located between your legs, and run from your pubic bone at the front to the base of your spine at the back. They are in the shape of a sling and hold your bladder and urethra in place. They give you control over your bladder and are used to urinate. As you get older, your pelvic floor muscles get weaker. Women who have had children may also find they have weaker pelvic floor muscles, which can cause problems such as urinary incontinence (being unable to control when you pass urine) and reduced sensitivity (feeling) during sex. Doing pelvic floor exercises can help to keep your pelvic muscles strong. Both men and women can do pelvic floor exercises.

You can feel your pelvic floor muscles if you try to stop the flow of urine when you go to the toilet. To strengthen them, sit comfortably and squeeze the muscles 10–15 times in a row. Avoid holding your breath, or tightening your stomach, buttock or thigh muscles at the same time. When you get used to doing pelvic floor exercises, you can try holding each squeeze for a few seconds. Every week you can add more squeezes, but be careful not to overdo it, and always have a rest in between sets of squeezes. After a few months you should start to notice the results. Any incontinence should improve, as well as the sensitivity you experience during sex. You should carry on doing the exercises, even when you notice them starting to work.

How many Caesarean sections can one have?

There is no limit to the number of Caesarean sections you can have. However, the risk of some complications during pregnancy and birth is higher if you have had one or more Caesarean sections before. This is because having a Caesarean section produces a scar on your womb where the incision is made. The risk of complications doesn't necessarily get higher if you've had more than one Caesarean section. The complications include *placenta praevia*, when the baby's placenta attaches near or on the opening of your cervix, and *placenta accreta*, when the baby's placenta grows in the lining of your womb and into or through the muscle in your womb. Both of these conditions increase your risk of complications when giving birth such as serious bleeding, shock and emergency hysterectomy.

It may not be possible to have a vaginal birth if you have had one or more Caesarean sections in the past. This is because there is a chance that your womb could tear along the scars from any previous Caesarean sections (a uterine rupture) when you give birth vaginally.

If you have had a Caesarean section previously, your doctor should be prepared to carry out an emergency Caesarean section if complications develop during a vaginal birth.

Did You Know... Babies are born with 300 bones, but by adulthood the number is reduced to 206. The reason for this is that many of the bones of children are composed of smaller component bones that are not yet fused, like those in the skull. This makes it easier for the baby to pass through the birth canal. The bones harden and fuse as the children grow.

Why aren't separate measles, mumps and rubella jabs available on the NHS?

The MMR jab contains three separate vaccines in one injection, and protects children against measles, mumps and rubella. Independent expert groups from all around the world, including the World Health Organization and the UK Department of Health, agree that the MMR vaccination is preferable to having three separate injections. There is no evidence to suggest that separate vaccines are safer than the MMR vaccination, and having single vaccines could put your child at risk of catching the diseases she has not yet been vaccinated against in the gaps between vaccines. As the MMR vaccination is the safest, most effective way of protecting children against measles, mumps and rubella, the NHS does not offer separate vaccines.

Questions about the MMR jab's safety arose when a report was published claiming a link between the MMR jab and autism and/or inflammatory bowel disease, but since then many studies investigating this claim have found no link between the MMR vaccine and these conditions, and have also found that this initial research was seriously flawed in both its technique and its ethics. Its author has since been removed from the medical register.

When should I start giving my baby solid food, and what should I give her?

For the first six months, breastmilk – and/or formula – provides all the nutrients and fluids that your baby needs. The UK Department of Health recommends that solid food should not be introduced before a baby is six months of age. Also, after six months you should continue breastfeeding and/or giving your baby breastmilk substitute alongside solid food up to two years of age, or beyond.

Soft, runny foods should be given when weaning your baby because babies are not able to chew at this age. Start with baby rice, cooked and puréed vegetables such as carrot, butternut squash or avocado, or fruit such as banana or stewed eating apple. As your baby gets older, you can slowly introduce textured foods such as lumpy purées, rice cakes or breadsticks, which will teach her to chew. Meat, fish, dairy products and pulses are all excellent sources of iron and protein, and are important for sustaining your baby's rapid rate of growth and development.

Commercial baby food products can be convenient and you may want to use them from time to time. However, you should not rely on them. Wherever possible, you should give your child fresh food; home-cooked meals are inexpensive and you know exactly what has gone into them. Avoid giving your baby gluten, salt, shellfish, nuts and honey.

My baby was born with a condition called hypospadias. He has to have an operation but I don't really understand it – can you explain why he needs it and what happens?

Hypospadias is the most commonly seen genital abnormality that boys are born with, and it can run in families. All that occurs in this condition is that instead of the opening through which pee comes being at the end, or tip, of the penis, it can be anywhere along the shaft instead. In 90 per cent of cases the abnormality is mild and the opening is found very close to where it should be. Surgery involves correcting the defect so that the end of the urethra is found back at the end of the penis. It is usually done when a baby is one year old.

Did You Know… A baby's head is one-quarter of its total length, but by age 25 will only be one-eighth of a person's total length. Our heads don't change size as drastically as the rest of our body: legs and torso will lengthen, but our head won't get much longer.

My baby girl is two weeks old and seems to be making milk! She is producing a white discharge from her nipples and I'm really worried about it. Has she got some terrible problem?

No, this sounds like something very straightforward but which can be a bit alarming for new mothers. You are right to say that she seems to be producing milk – she almost certainly is. It used to be called 'witch's milk' (back in less enlightened days!) and is simply the result of hormones from the mother affecting the baby at the time of the birth, or in the milk the baby is drinking. It can occur in babies of either sex, and is in no way detrimental to their health.

No treatment is needed and the milk production usually disappears in a few weeks. Interestingly, any woman – or man – can be made to produce breastmilk if they are given the correct hormone cocktail at almost any time in their lives.

I have recently found out I am pregnant. I am very fit and train rigorously four times a week, doing weights and cardio work. Can I keep up this regime during my pregnancy, or is it dangerous? I have also been told I shouldn't cycle or do stomach muscle exercises. Is this correct?

I think the most salient phrase to use here is 'common sense'. Although there is only a very rarely reported link between exercise and miscarriage, you should take things a little easier to allow your body a chance to adapt to the massive changes that occur during pregnancy. Exercises like swimming, light jogging and light weights should be fine, as long as you are getting enough rest and eating healthily.

Cycling is not a problem as such provided it is not too strenuous, and gentle sit-ups or leg raises are OK, too, provided you feel no discomfort when doing them.

My period is late and I have been trying to get pregnant. I'm due to take a long-distance flight very soon and want to know whether it is safe to fly and if the radiation levels in the plane could have an effect on my pregnancy?

Flying is certainly not advised against in an uncomplicated pregnancy, so provided that you and the baby are in good health prior to take-off, then flying is not likely to pose significant health risks.

Most of the studies on pregnancy and air travel have been done on female flight attendants. One study did show that there was a slight increase in miscarriage during the first three months of pregnancy, but this was for the flight attendants who worked a greater number of hours, flying on average 74 hours per month.

Concerns have been raised with in-flight radiation as some studies have shown a slight increase in potential problems, but these were mainly for frequent long-distance flyers. In your case this single flight is unlikely to be detrimental to your pregnancy.

The only restrictions for pregnant women come at the later stages of pregnancy, when some airlines do not permit women who are more than 36 weeks pregnant to fly, to avoid an in-flight delivery.

Amazing Human Abilities

1) Supertasters

Supertasters are people with a far heightened sense of taste. They have extra tastebuds on their tongues. Of the five types of taste (sweet, sour, salty, bitter and umami), supertasters generally find bitterness to be the most perceptible, and so will often dislike bitter foods such as Brussels sprouts, cabbage, coffee and grapefruit juice.

2) Perfect pitch

People with perfect pitch are capable of identifying and reproducing a note at the correct pitch without needing a known reference. In other words, they can actually remember pitches and reproduce them correctly. Opinions vary as to whether absolute pitch is genetic or a learned ability. Around 3 per cent of the general population in the US and Europe have perfect pitch, but in musicians this goes up to 8 per cent. More impressive is the fact that in music conservatories in Japan, about 70 per cent of musicians have perfect pitch. It's also more common in those who are blind from birth, or have autism.

3) Tetrachromacy

This is the ability to see light from four distinct sources. True tetrachromacy in humans is very rare – it's thought that only two possible tetrachromats have ever been identified. Humans are normally trichromats, having three types of cone cells that receive light from either the red, green or blue part of the spectrum. Tetrachromats have an extra type of cone between red and green (in the orange range) that allows them to see a far greater range of the spectrum. Interestingly, colour-blindness in men may be inherited from women with tetrachromacy.

4) Echolocation

Bats fly around in the dark using echolocation. They emit a sound, wait for the echo to return, and use that to work out how far away an object is. Amazingly, humans are capable of using echolocation, too. Blind people have learned to master it, although it takes time and a heightened sensitivity to reflected sound.

5) Genetic Chimerism

Homer, in his great work *The Iliad*, describes a creature with body parts from different animals: a chimera. This is how we get the term chimerism. Genetic chimerism in humans occurs when two fertilized eggs or embryos fuse together early in pregnancy. Each carries a copy of its parents' DNA and thus a distinct genetic profile. When these merge, each population of cells retains its genetic character and the resulting single embryo becomes a mixture of both. Bafflingly, a human chimera is his or her own twin! Chimeric people also have immune systems that make them tolerant to both of their genetically distinct populations of cells, meaning that a chimera has a much wider array of people to choose from should he or she need an organ transplant.

6) Synaesthesia

This means experiencing sensations in unusual ways, like associating numbers or letters with certain colours, or hearing a specific word which triggers a particular sensation of taste. It's often genetic and the grapheme form (letters, numbers or other symbols) is the most common. Other synaesthetes can experience special-sequence synaesthesia (where dates have a precise location in space), ordinal-linguistic personification (when numbers have personalities), or sound-to-colour synaesthesia (where tones are perceived as colours). Studies suggest around 1 in 23 people have some form of synaesthesia.

7) Mental Calculators

While there are many trained people who can calculate with large numbers in their head extremely fast, the untrained ability of autistic savants is the most impressive. They are adept at performing hugely complex mental calculations. There are fewer than 100 recognized prodigious savants in the world, and even fewer savants who are capable of using mental calculation techniques. Research has found they have a blood flow to the part of their brains responsible for mathematical calculations six to seven times the normal rate.

8) Eidetic Memory

Otherwise known as a photographic memory or total recall, people with this ability can recall sounds, images or objects with extreme accuracy. Examples include the effort of one man who recited from memory the first 100,000 decimal places of pi and another, the inspiration for the character of Raymond Babbitt in the film *Rain Man*, who could recall some 12,000 books from memory. Despite the promises of certain courses advertised on the Internet, one cannot become an *eidetiker* through practice.

9) Immortal Cells

There is only one known case of a person having immortal cells, or cells that can divide indefinitely outside the human body. In 1951 woman called Henrietta Lacks died from cervical cancer, aged 31. A surgeon took a tissue sample from her tumour and it was propagated into an immortal cell line known as the HeLa cell line. These cells have an active version of the telomerase enzyme, involved in cell-repairing and cell-ageing, and they also proliferate abnormally fast. HeLa cells were used by Jonas Salk to develop the polio vaccine, and have been used in researching cancer, AIDS, the effects of radiation and toxic substances, and for mapping genes, ever since. Interestingly, there are more HeLa cells alive today than when Henrietta Lacks was alive.

Is it true that you can get varicose veins on the vulva? I'm pregnant and am getting some pains in that area, which my doctor said could be due to these veins.

You can get vulval varicose veins and they tend to cause aching and irritation, which can be severe. They become more common as pregnancy progresses. They are caused by a similar process to varicose veins in the legs, but in this case the enlarging womb obstructs blood flow back to the heart, causing increased pressure in the veins that can damage them and cause them to become varicose. The body can easily cope without these veins, as you have deeper veins that do the same job, but the varicose veins are unsightly and often uncomfortable.

Swelling of the vulva and increased blood supply to the area is a feature of pregnancy and this may be a cause of your symptoms, as could common infections like thrush. They should disappear after the baby is born.

Did You Know... During pregnancy, the average woman's uterus expands up to 500 times its normal size.

How soon can I do a pregnancy test?

Pregnancy tests are designed to detect the presence of the pregnancy hormone human chorionic gonadotrophin (HCG). During pregnancy the amount of HCG in your body rises rapidly in the early stages, and a home pregnancy test can detect this in your urine. You can do a test from the day that your period was due. Counting the number of days from the first day of your last period until the day before your next period is due to start will give you your usual cycle length. If you don't know when your next period is due, wait at least 19 days after you last had unprotected sex before testing. If the result is negative but you are not convinced, then wait another three days before testing again. You may have conceived later than you thought and there might not have been enough HCG in your urine to be picked up by the first test.

There are other clues to possible pregnancy. Certain symptoms such as enlarged or tingling breasts, nausea, dizziness, a metallic taste in your mouth and a feeling that your period is about to start are all typical in the early stages of pregnancy, but not all women get these symptoms.

How long does it usually take to get pregnant?

It is impossible to say exactly how long it will take a couple to get pregnant, as many factors such as age, general and reproductive health, and when you have intercourse can all play their part. Some couples conceive within the first month of trying, while others take much longer. Generally doctors would not consider investigating you for fertility issues until you had been trying unsuccessfully to get pregnant for a year. Around 9 out of 10 couples conceive within a year of trying, and around half of those who have been trying unsuccessfully for a year will conceive the following year.

For a woman aged 20–25, the chances of conceiving are 25 per cent for each cycle. For a woman aged 30–35, the chances of conceiving are 15 per cent for each cycle. It will usually take a couple in their twenties an average of five cycles to conceive, and it can take a couple in their thirties around nine cycles to conceive.

A midwife told me that babies all have the same colour eyes at birth. This can't be true, can it?

It is. Babies are always born with blue eyes. It's true that the genes inherited from your parents determine the colour of your eyes, but at birth most babies appear to have blue eyes. The reason is to do with the pigment melanin, which in a newborn's eyes often still needs time to be fully deposited or to be darkened by exposure to ultraviolet light, revealing the baby's true eye colour.

Is it dangerous to get flu when you are pregnant? There are always outbreaks, and with swine flu around I am worried.

Flu is caused by a virus, which comes in many different strains and severities. Some viruses can cross the placenta and infect a developing baby, like rubella and varicella, but flu is not one of them. A bout of flu may make *you* feel rough, but it won't affect your baby in any way. If you do catch it then take paracetamol and rest. Avoid aspirin, which can affect your baby's heart and circulatory system. I would always advise you to consult a doctor if you have an unexplained high fever during pregnancy: certain bacteria such as listeria can cause miscarriage or premature birth, and should be treated with antibiotics.

Did You Know... Babies breathe much faster than adults – 30 to 50 times a minute compared to an adult's 15 to 20 times a minute.

Why do pregnant women get morning sickness? I get it all day long and don't think I can cope any more. What can I do?

Morning sickness is most common during the first three months of pregnancy. The exact cause is unknown, but it's thought to be exacerbated by rising levels of the hormone human chorionic gonadotrophin (HCG), which is produced in large quantities up until 12 to 14 weeks. Other hormones like oestrogen and thyroxine may also be responsible. Be reassured that for most women it doesn't continue much beyond week 12, however.

If you are tired, hungry or stressed the nausea can be worse, and if you are having a multiple pregnancy then you will have higher levels of pregnancy hormones, and may get more severe sickness, too.

It's probably the most common condition of early pregnancy, but the term 'morning sickness' is misleading as most sufferers get it throughout the day and into the evening. A very severe form exists called *hyperemesis gravidarum*, which causes sufferers to vomit many times a day and makes them unable to eat and drink without vomiting. It can require hospitalization to treat.

Because it is such a normal part of pregnancy it can be difficult to treat. Make sure you are getting enough rest and avoid stress, and try eating little and often. Work out which foods suit you and which may make your symptoms worse. Remember to keep well hydrated. Vitamin B_6-rich foods or a good quality vitamin B complex supplement may also be helpful, as one study found that B_6 supplements may help reduce nausea in pregnancy, although there was no effect on vomiting. The Food Standards Agency recommends that no more than 10mg of B_6 should be taken each day as a supplement. Ginger, peppermint, lemon balm and chamomile tea have also been recommended.

I have an agonizing pain in my tailbone, all round my pelvis, over my pubic area and down my thighs. I'm seven months pregnant and want to know what I can do about it?

You are describing a condition called *diastasis symphisis pubis*, for which I'm afraid there is no known cure. It may be present up to and for a few weeks beyond the birth, but almost always improves after then. Warm baths, physiotherapy and paracetamol can all help to relieve the pain.

The dreaded chickenpox is currently infecting my two young kids. My friends are nervous to come round as they say they might catch shingles from them. Is this possible?

It is not possible to catch shingles from chickenpox. Your friends could catch chickenpox from your children, but only if they have no immunity to it already (from having had chickenpox or having gained immunity from their mother when they were in the womb). Your children are OK to play with anyone other than pregnant mothers who have never had the infection, newborn babies, and people with very weakened immune systems.

Shingles isn't actually caught from anyone: it's an old chickenpox virus that has been living in the nerve root in the spine and gets reactivated, causing the classic painful blistering rash.

Did You Know... A baby born before 37 weeks of pregnancy is considered a premature baby. Every day, over 1,300 babies are born prematurely in the United States. The largest surviving baby ever born weighed 6.7 kg (14 lb 13 oz) and was nearly 58.42 cm (23 inches) in length.

Can you tell if a baby in the womb is a boy or a girl by how it is lying? I was always told that if 'carrying high' then it's a girl, if low, a boy.

The ability to predict the future is something humans have been trying to do since we first gained self-awareness. From the outcomes of battles to the sex of an unborn child, many wild claims have been made. The Oracle at Delphi in ancient Greece and the sixteenth century seer Nostradamus are famous for their predictive powers. There is clearly something appealing about gender-predicting techniques, because there are dozens of them: the heart-rate method, the ring-swing method, the 'how sick are you?' approach, not to mention determinations based on keys, acne, dreams, skin tone and food cravings.

The most popular of all is the 'high or low' determination that you describe. And it's not just 'high or low'. There's also the belief that 'carrying wide' indicates a girl, and 'carrying narrow' means it's a boy.

So is it right? Well, yes, 50 per cent of the time. Lots of people would swear by these methods; but when there's always a 50/50 chance of being right, you're going to find lots of correct predictions and, therefore, many convinced people.

It's not the gender of the baby that determines its position in the womb, it's the strength and tone of the mother's abdominal muscles. The tighter a woman's abdominal muscles (either due to age or fitness level), the higher the bump rides. An older woman or one who's had her abdominal muscles loosened by prior pregnancies will usually carry lower.

The only reasonably accurate way to know the gender of a baby is via amniocentesis or an ultrasound scan, but even ultrasound can fail if your baby has his or her legs crossed!

NB: In the last few years some at-home gender-prediction tests have become available, sold with a baffling description of the 'scientific proof' backing them. They're supposed to predict gender accurately based on the composition of the woman's urine. In truth there is little evidence to substantiate their claims.

PREGNANCY TOP TIPS

1. Do not smoke! Stop before you get pregnant and stay stopped. There is nothing beneficial in smoking and it can cause many problems.

2. Drink a maximum of just one or two units of alcohol once or twice a week. I would advise women not to drink alcohol at all in the first three months of pregnancy, because of the increased risk of miscarriage.

3. Eat a balanced diet with plenty of fruit and vegetables.

4. Take a folic acid supplement, starting from when you are trying to conceive up until the 12th week of pregnancy.

5. Avoid vitamin A supplements, as they can harm your baby.

6. Try to avoid eating liver (e.g. in paté), ripened soft cheeses and raw eggs.

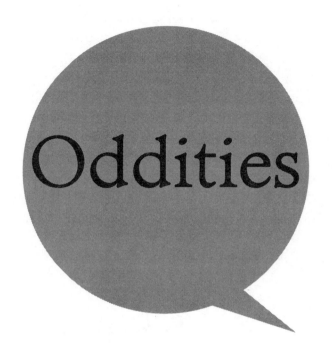

Why do your hands and feet go wrinkly in the bath, but not the rest of you?

The outer layer of your skin, the epidermis, produces an oily substance called sebum that keeps water off our skins, but after a long period underwater, the sebum is washed off and the skin starts to absorb water, causing the epidermis to expand and therefore have a greater surface area. Being attached to the tissue below, it wrinkles to compensate for the greater surface area. Because there is less room on your fingers and toes, the skin appears more wrinkled. It doesn't occur elsewhere on your body as the skin is better able to cope with a degree of swelling.

Will sitting too close to the TV ruin your vision and give you square eyes?

This is one of the great myths. Being close to the TV won't ruin your eyesight, but sitting less than 1.5 metres (about 5 ft) from the set may tire the muscles that focus the lens of the eye, resulting in eyestrain and tired eyes that burn and water. Make sure you sit further than 1.5 metres from the TV set and have enough light in the room, and give your eyes a break by refocusing your gaze during commercial breaks, and no long-term damage will occur.

Did You Know... The colder the room you sleep in, the better the chances are that you'll have a bad dream. It isn't entirely clear to scientists why this is the case, but if you would rather not have nightmares you might want to keep yourself a little toastier at night.

What is colour blindness?

Colour blindness is the reduced ability to distinguish between certain colours. It's usually inherited and is more common in men, affecting about one in 20. Far fewer women – around one in 200 – are affected. This is because many of the genes involved in colour vision are located on the X chromosome. Males have only one X chromosome, while females have two, making the probability of having two defective genes more unlikely.

The most common form causes an inability to differentiate between the colours red and green. In some men other colours may be involved, but only rarely is all colour vision lost so that the person sees only in black and white.

The retina of the eye has colour-detecting vision cells, called cones, which are necessary to see colour properly. There are three types of cone cell, detecting red, blue or green light. If one or more of these types of cells is faulty, then colour blindness results.

Sometimes colour blindness can occur because of diseases such as macular degeneration or as a side-effect of certain medicines.

Colour blindness is classed by some as a mild disability; however, in certain situations colour-blind individuals have an advantage over those with normal colour vision. There are some studies that concluded that colour-blind individuals are better at penetrating certain colour camouflages, and it has been suggested that this may be the evolutionary explanation for the surprisingly high frequency of congenital red–green colour blindness.

I was always told that if you swallowed your chewing gum it would stay in you for seven years. Is this true?

No. If swallowed, the average piece of gum will be expelled in the stool a few days later. Gum is not digested and takes slightly longer to be expelled than food, which is digested and passes through the intestinal tract in about 24 hours. Only if a very small child swallows a huge wad of gum is there any danger of the gum causing an intestinal obstruction. In that case it could take much longer to be expelled, but nothing close to seven years. In severe cases this could lead to distension of the intestines and severe abdominal cramps, and may require surgery to remove the obstruction.

Why are only a few people left-handed? Is this due to a malfunction of the brain?

About 4 per cent of the population is left-handed, and there are more left-handed males than females. In past times left-handers were considered suspicious, shifty and clumsy people. It's where we get the word 'sinister' from – the Latin word for left is *sinistra*.

Today most researchers agree that hand preference is produced by biological and, most likely, genetic causes. The two most widely accepted theories claim that evolutionary natural selection produced a majority of individuals with speech and language control in the left hemisphere of the brain. Because the left hemisphere also controls the movements of the right hand – and notably the movements needed to produce written language – millennia of evolutionary development resulted in a population of humans biased genetically toward individuals with left hemisphere speech/language and right-hand preference.

The idea of handedness is intriguing because external cultural and societal pressures can influence it. Also, hand preference does not appear to be a characteristic of animals; it seems to be exclusive to humans

While there is good evidence that left-handedness is more common in people with reading disabilities, stuttering and poor coordination, some of these problems stem from the fact that traditionally many left-handers were made to use their less coordinated right hand. In fact there is an impressive list of left-handed leaders, artists and sportspeople including Queen Victoria, Harry Truman, Michelangelo, Leonardo da Vinci, Paul McCartney, Judy Garland and Pablo Picasso.

As some say – perhaps left-handed people are the only people in their right minds? For the record, I'm left-handed.

Did You Know... Right-handed people live, on average, nine years longer than left-handed people. This doesn't have a genetic basis, but is largely due to the fact that a majority of the machines and tools we use on a daily basis are designed for those who are right-handed, making them somewhat dangerous for lefties to use and resulting in thousands of accidents and deaths each year.

What is the best hangover cure?

There is no scientific evidence of an effective cure or method for preventing hangovers, despite many trials being carried out on both traditional and complementary medicines. As a general rule the darker the alcohol the worse the hangover, so vodka and gin tend not to have as bad a day-after effect as brandy or whisky. All alcohol dehydrates, which will make everything worse, so drinking water every other drink should help a bit.

My mother used to tell me never to go to bed with wet hair, as I would catch a cold, and always to wear a hat in cold weather as we lose heat most through our heads. Is this really true?

No more heat is lost through the head than from any other uncovered part of the body. This can easily been seen using an infrared heat detecting camera. Being cold and wet does not cause colds. You also won't catch a cold from going outside without your coat, and you won't catch cold from going to bed with a wet head. Colds are caused by viruses so you need to be exposed to the virus in order to get one.

There are more suicides at Christmas. True?

While the combined stresses of family dysfunction, exacerbations in loneliness and depression over the cold, dark winter months are commonly thought to increase the number of suicides, there is no good evidence to suggest a peak in suicides at Christmas time. People are actually not more likely to commit suicide in the dark winter months – globally, suicides peak in warmer months, according to research.

Why did the nurse take my flowers away at night when I was in hospital?

There are many old wives' tales concerning hospital flowers. One says that if you put red and white flowers together in a vase in a hospital room, a person in the surrounding ward will die. Another common legend goes that patients should always leave flower arrangements behind in the hospital room when they're discharged; if they bring the flowers home, they'll end up right back in the hospital.

These are not the reason the nurse took your flowers away, however (I hope). Some people think that flowers are bad for hospital rooms because they suck oxygen out of the air. And people need their oxygen, especially sick ones! On the surface, the oxygen-depletion myth is true in part. Whilst plants typically absorb carbon dioxide and emit oxygen during the day, at night they absorb more oxygen than they produce, and they emit carbon dioxide. But overall flowers add far more oxygen to a hospital room than they use. In the daytime plants emit 10 times more oxygen than they use up at night, so a hospital room with flowers in it will actually end up more oxygenated than one without. It would actually make far more sense to ban visitors, who use up far more oxygen than a vase of flowers.

In short, taking your flowers away was silly. At least one study has shown that having flowers in a hospital room makes patients feel better. A 2008 study in the *Journal of the American Society for Horticultural Science* revealed that patients in hospital rooms containing flowers or potted plants used less pain medication and had lower blood pressure than patients in rooms without them

The reason flowers are often banned outright from intensive care units is due to bacteria. The water in a vase of cut flowers can carry harmful bacteria, although this bacterial source has never actually led to a case of patient illness.

Did You Know... Humans are the only animals to produce emotional tears. In the animal world, humans are the biggest cry-babies, being the only animals who cry because they've had a bad day, lost a loved one, or just don't feel good.

Will going swimming after eating give you cramp?

This is a much-spread myth. No one is quite sure when or why parents began telling their children to wait an hour after eating before going swimming. It seems to have been believed that, after eating, most of the available blood in one's body would flood to the stomach to help with digestion and so would not be available to supply the limbs adequately when swimming, resulting in cramp.

It's true that blood flows to our stomachs after we eat a big meal. While there it gets busy absorbing nutrients, leaving less of the stuff available to deliver oxygen and remove waste products elsewhere in the body. But the truth is that we have enough blood to keep all of our other parts running just fine after a meal. In fact, some competitive swimmers eat something immediately before a big meet to give themselves the energy they need to perform well.

Top 10 Unusual Psychological Disorders

1) Trichotillomania

An impulse-control disorder or form of self-injury characterized by the repeated pulling out of hair, be it from the scalp, eyelashes, face, nose, eyebrows or pubic region, sometimes causing noticeable bald patches. It can resemble a habit, an addiction, a tic disorder or an obsessive-compulsive disorder. It often begins during the teenage years and can be triggered by depression or stress.

2) Oniomania

A compulsive desire to shop, also known as compulsive shopping, compulsive buying, shopping addiction or shopaholism. Sufferers often experience moods of satisfaction when they are in the process of purchasing, which seems to give their life meaning while letting them forget about their sorrows. Unfortunately the feeling of personal reward quickly withers, and so to compensate the addicted person goes shopping again and again. In some cases they may hide or destroy the purchases due to shame and embarrassment.

3) Nymphomania

Well known to the public, nymphomania is an uncontrollable urge in women to have sex. Now more commonly known as hypersexuality, it makes sufferers unable to control their sexual impulses, which can involve the entire spectrum of sexual fantasy or behaviour. Eventually the sexual activity interferes with the person's social, vocational or marital life, which begins to deteriorate. When a man has this same kind of problem, it is called satyriasis.

4) Dissociative Identity Disorder

Formerly known as multiple personality syndrome, this is a condition in which a single person displays multiple distinct identities or personalities, each with its own pattern of perceiving and interacting with the environment. The diagnosis requires that at least two personalities routinely take control of the individual's behaviour with an associated memory loss that goes beyond normal forgetfulness. Despite the fact that 40,000 cases were diagnosed from 1985 to 1995, some therapists consider it not to exist at all.

5) Piblokto

Also known as Pibloktoq or Arctic Hysteria, this is a condition exclusive to societies living within the Arctic Circle. Most often seen during the winter months and more common in women, its symptoms include intense hysteria (screaming, uncontrolled wild behaviour), depression, coprophagia (eating poo), insensitivity to extreme cold (such as running around in the snow naked), echolalia (senseless repetition of overheard words) and more. It may be linked to vitamin A toxicity because the native diet provides rich sources of vitamin A.

6) Coprolalia

Involuntary swearing or utterance of obscene words or socially inappropriate and derogatory remarks (not to be confused with Tourette Syndrome, which is identified by both physical and vocal tics). Involuntary outbursts such as racial or ethnic slurs in the company of those most offended by such remarks are unavoidable, though the comments do not necessarily reflect the thoughts or opinions of the affected person.

Related disorders include copropraxia: performing obscene or forbidden gestures, and coprographia: making obscene writings or drawings.

7) Jumping Frenchmen of Maine

A rare disorder first described in 1878. An individual with this disorder has a genetic mutation that prevents 'exciting' signals in the nervous system from being regulated, which causes a number of bizarre irregularities in their startle response. This means that an event which might only startle an unaffected person will result in an extended, grossly exaggerated response from a 'jumper', including crying out, flailing limbs, twitching and sometimes convulsions. Another curious abnormality caused by this disorder is a sufferer's automatic reflex to obey any order that is delivered suddenly. For example, the sudden barked command to throw an object will result in just that happening, whether a jumper wanted to or not. Similarly if they are told to hit a person, they will, even if it is a loved one.

8) Depersonalization

A strange disorder in which the sufferer feels that they are living in a dream world. Some describe it as a feeling of watching oneself act, while having no control. It can be recreated as a desired effect of recreational drugs, but the term usually refers to the severe form found in anxiety and panic attacks. Also it can cause sufferers to lose awareness of their own identity, giving the condition its name.

9) Cotard Delusion

A rare psychiatric disorder in which a person holds a delusional belief that he or she is dead, does not exist, is putrefying or has lost blood or internal organs. Rarely, it can include delusions of immortality. It is named after Jules Cotard, a French neurologist who first described the condition in 1880, which he called 'le délire de négation' – negation delirium.

10) Zoosadism

Refers to pleasure, sometimes sexual, derived from cruelty to animals. Zoosadism is part of the triad of behaviours that are a precursor to sociopathic behaviour. There have been many cases of 'horse-ripping' that have sexual connotations, and in general, the link between sadistic sexual acts with animals and sadistic practices with humans or lust murders has been heavily researched and identified. 36 per cent of murderers claim to have tortured animals in their childhood, with some of them also practising bestiality. 46 per cent of them reported that they had abused animals during adolescence, and many sexual murderers showed an interest in zoosexual acts.

If you step on a rusty nail, will you really get tetanus?

This legend is partly true: stepping on a rusty nail has the potential to cause tetanus. But so can a perfectly clean nail, a sewing needle or a scratch from an animal.

Tetanus is caused by bacteria known as *Clostridium tetani*, which is commonly found in soil, dust and animal faeces. Because of its presence in soil and manure, gardeners and others who work in agriculture are particularly at risk of exposure to these bacteria; indeed, some farmers may even have it on their skin.

When in the soil or on the skin, *C. tetani* isn't dangerous, because it can only reproduce in an oxygen-deprived setting. A puncture wound, such as one that might occur from stepping on a nail, can provide that breeding ground. Within the wound, *C. tetani* releases a neurotoxin known as tetanospasmin, which may be the second most powerful toxin after botulinum. Rust is not in and of itself a *C. tetani* carrier; rather, the thinking goes that if the nail has been outside long enough to get rusty, then it's probably been exposed to soils containing the bacteria. The crevices of the rust give the soil a place to hide, and the deep puncture wound gives the *C. tetani* a place to do its work.

Do nails and hair continue growth after death? You always hear stories of coffins being open and the person's nails being longer, but does it really happen – and if so, how?

Nails and hair do *not* continue to grow after we die – but they can appear longer. This is because the skin dehydrates and pulls back from the nail beds and scalp, exposing more of the hair and nails. But it's not growing. Once dead, we stay dead. All of us.

Why are bogies green?

People often ask me if I ever find anything truly yucky or if I am desensitized to it all by now. The answer is yes, I do still find a few things yucky: feet, followed closely by snot. Writing the answer to this question is making me squirm already. Your snot shouldn't really be green all the time – usually only when you have a cold. The snot of a healthy person is typically white or clear, although during the early stages of a cold it can still be clear, just very copious! Brown and brown-grey mucus is common in smokers and is caused by the cigarette tar sticking to the mucus. Rusty coloured or blood-spotted phlegm can be a sign of more serious illness such as pneumonia or bleeding from an airway, which can be a sign of cancer. And then there is the green variety, nearly always present during an infection. It's all to do with the immune processes that go on during a cold. The mucous in your nose acts as a barrier against germs, dust and other noxious substances that we breathe in by the bucketful each day. These all get trapped in the mucous and, if necessary, are destroyed by our immune system. Cells called neutrophils fight invading pathogens by engulfing and destroying them using digestive enzymes. Some of these enzymes, such as lactoferrin, require iron for their optimum activity. One such enzyme, called myeloperoxidase, produces the antiseptic chemical hypochlorous acid, the same type of bleach commonly used to sanitize swimming pools. Interestingly, it is similar iron-containing enzymes in wasabi that make it green, too. Funnily enough I don't like wasabi either! So the colour of your snot during a cold is green because of the iron used to fight the cold – ferrous iron compounds are green.

I'm really ticklish if anyone touches me, but why can't I tickle myself?

Even the most ticklish among us do not have the ability to tickle ourselves. The reason behind this is that your brain predicts the tickle from information it already has, like how your fingers are moving. Because it knows and can feel where the tickle is coming from, your brain doesn't respond in the same way as if someone else is doing the tickling.

Did You Know... Your ears secrete more earwax when you are afraid than when you aren't. The chemicals and hormones released when you are afraid could be having unseen effects on your body, in the form of earwax. Studies have suggested that fear causes the ears to produce more of the sticky substance, though the reasons are not yet clear.

Is there such a thing as a true hermaphrodite? If so, could they get themselves pregnant?

A true hermaphrodite should more correctly be called an intersex person. Strictly defined, intersexuality is when someone's genitals are either ambiguous or combine male and female elements. It's almost always the result of a genetic disorder. Gonads (testicles or ovaries) can form with a combination of male and female parts, women can be born without a vagina, and some people can be born with both a penis and a vagina. One especially unusual type of intersex person is known as a *chimera*, which results when male and female embryos meld together genetically to form one individual.

Could an intersex person get him-/herself pregnant? Well, the necessities for pregnancy are a sperm, an egg, a way for the two to meet, a uterus for foetal development, and the proper hormone levels. Most intersex people are unable to provide at least one of these critical bits. Functioning ovaries are fairly common in the intersexed, but functioning testes are rarer, though not completely unknown. Functioning ovaries *and* functioning testes, however, plus functioning everything else, is extremely rare. In intersexuality you typically get a mix of male and female pieces, not two complete sets.

I remember a lecturer telling us that we only breathe through one nostril at a time. Is this true, and why then do we have two?

Amazingly, it is true and was first noted and explained in 1895 by a chap called Kayser, a German rhinologist from Breslau. He found that humans have a nasal cycle determined by the congestion and decongestion of the veins lining the nose. The veins form a spongy tissue, similar to erectile tissue in the penis, which is particularly well developed at the front of the nasal septum and the inferior turbinates (lower nasal passages).

During the day they switch over approximately every four hours or so, the engorged vessels blocking first one nostril and then the other.

This means that we do not usually breathe equally using both nostrils: one nostril is always more open and has a greater amount of airflow.

Not everyone's nose does this, however. It is present in about 85 per cent of people and can be affected by position (for example whether you are sitting upright or lying down), allergies and upper respiratory infections.

Eastern cultures have known about this far longer than we have in the West, as it is central to various breathing practices such as pranayama in yoga and also in various systems of alternative medicine.

Did You Know... Your body gives off enough heat in 30 minutes to bring nearly 2 litres (half a gallon) of water to a boil. If you've seen *The Matrix*, you are aware of the energy potentially generated by the human body. Our bodies expend a large amount of calories keeping us at a steady 37°C (98.6°F), enough to boil water or even cook pasta.

Why is coconut water known as the 'water of life'?

Many cultures call coconut water the 'water of life', and it seems they are not far wrong. It seems amazing, but coconut water has the same level of electrolytic balance as our blood. It has indeed been used in emergency cases as an intravenous hydration fluid when there is a lack of standard IV fluid. It's high in potassium, chloride and calcium, and could actually be used in situations requiring increases in these electrolytes. It's a close substitute for blood plasma as it is sterile, cool, easily absorbed by the body and does not destroy red blood cells.

Why do I sneeze when I enter into sunlight from a darkened room?

Usually, sneezing is the mechanism by which the body rids itself of irritants. But some people sneeze for a different reason. This is known as the photic sneeze reflex, and causes sneezing to occur on sudden exposure to bright light. This is also referred to as sun sneezing, photogenic sneezing, the photosternutatory reflex, and being allergic to the sun. The most impressive name for it that I have found is the autosomal dominant compelling helio-ophthalmic outburst syndrome, or ACHOO for short. I kid you not. It affects 18–35 per cent of the human population.

The probable cause is a mix-up of nerve signals in the fifth cranial nerve, called the trigeminal nerve, which is responsible for sneezes and also for the optic nerve. Scientists call this phenomenon 'cross talk', and it simply means the interference between two closely related nerves. The trigeminal nerve consists of branches in several parts of the face, including parts of the eye and nose, including the sinus cavities, and the palate. When nerves are closely bundled, cross talk is common. The strong signals entering the optic nerve when it is exposed to bright light stimulate the trigeminal nerve as well, causing sneezing.

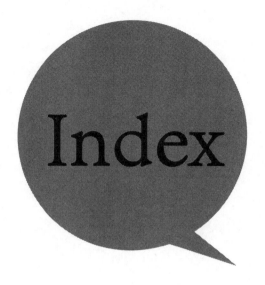

Index

NOTES

NOTES

NOTES

NOTES

NOTES

NOTES

NOTES

NOTES

NOTES

NOTES

NOTES

NOTES

NOTES